VOLUME 2

Musculoskeletal
Disorders
and
Congenital
Deformities

Atlas of the
Newborn

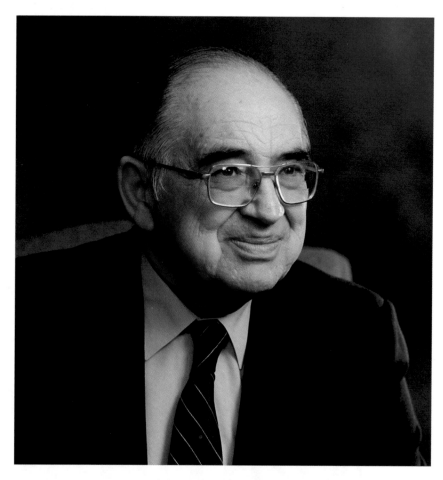

Arnold J. Rudolph, M.D.
(Deceased)
Professor of Pediatrics
Baylor Medical College
Houston, Texas

VOLUME 2

Musculoskeletal
Disorders
and
Congenital
Deformities

Atlas of the Newborn

Arnold J. Rudolph, M.D.
(Deceased)

1997

B.C. Decker Inc.
Hamilton • London

B.C. Decker Inc.
4 Hughson Street South
P.O. Box 620, L.C.D. 1
Hamilton, Ontario L8N 3K7
Tel: 905 522-7017
Fax: 905 522-7839
e-mail: info@bcdecker.com

Printed in Canada

9697989900/BP/987654321

ISBN 1-55009-032-1

Sales and distribution

United States
Blackwell Science Inc.
Commerce Place
350 Main Street
Malden, MA 02148
U.S.A.
Tel: 1-800-215-1000

Canada
Copp Clark Ltd.
200 Adelaide Street West
3rd Floor
Toronto, Ontario
Canada M5H 1W7
Tel: 416-597-1616
Fax: 416-597-1617

Japan
Igaku-Shoin Ltd.
Tokyo International P.O. Box 5063
1-28-36 Hongo, Bunkyo-ku
Tokyo 113, Japan
Tel: 3 3817 5680
Fax: 3 3815 7805

U.K., Europe, Scandinavia, Middle East
Blackwell Science Ltd.
c/o Marston Book Services Ltd.
P.O. Box 87
Oxford OX2 0DT
England
Tel: 44-1865-79115

Australia
Blackwell Science Pty, Ltd.
54 University Street
Carleton, Victoria 3053
Australia
Tel: 03 9347 0300
Fax: 03 9349 3016

Foreword

Sir William Osler stated, "There is no more difficult task in medicine than the art of observation." The late Arnold Jack Rudolph was an internationally renowned neonatologist, a teacher's teacher, and, above all, one who constantly reminded us about how much could be learned by simply observing, in his case, the newborn infant.

This color atlas of neonatology represents a distillation of more than 50 years of observing normal and abnormal newborn infants. The *Atlas* begins with a section on the placenta, its membranes, and the umbilical cord. Jack Rudolph delighted in giving a lecture entitled "Don't Make Mirth of the Afterbirth," in which he captivated audiences by showing them how much you could learn about the newborn infant from simply observing the placenta, its membranes, and the umbilical cord.

In a few more than 60 photomicrographs, we learn to read the placenta and gain insight into such disorders as intrauterine growth retardation, omphalitis, cytomegalic inclusion disease, congenital syphilis, and congenital neuroblastoma. Congenital abnormalities of every organ system are depicted along with the appearance of newborn infants who have been subjected in utero to a variety of different drugs, toxins, or chemicals. We also learn to appreciate the manifestations of birth trauma and abnormalities caused by abnormal intrauterine positioning.

More than 250 photographs are used to illustrate the field of neonatal dermatology. The collection of photographs used in this section is superior to that which I have seen in any other textbook or atlas of neonatology or dermatology; this section alone makes this reference a required addition to the library of any clinician interested in the care of infants and children. Photographs of the Kasabach-Merritt syndrome (cavernous hemangioma with thrombocytopenia), Klippel-Trénaunay syndrome, Turner's syndrome, Waardenburg's syndrome, neurocutaneous melanosis, mastocytosis (urticaria pigmentosa), and incon-tinentia pigmenti (Bloch-Sulzberger syndrome) are among the best that I have seen.

Cutaneous manifestations are associated with many perinatal infections. The varied manifestations of staphylococcal infection of the newborn are depicted vividly in photomicrographs of furunculosis, pyoderma, bullous impetigo, abscesses, parotitis, dacryocystitis, inastitis, cellulitis, omphalitis, and funisitis. Streptococcal cellulitis, *Haemophilus influenzae* cellulitis, and cutaneous manifestations of listeriosis all are depicted. There are numerous photomicrographs of congenital syphilis, showing the typical peripheral desquamative rash on the palms and soles, as well as other potential skin manifestations of congenital syphilis which may produce either vesicular, bullous, or ulcerative lesions. The various radiologic manifestations of congenital syphilis, including pneumonia alba, ascites, growth arrest lines, Wegner's sign, periostitis, and syphilitic osteochondritis, are depicted. Periostitis of the clavicle (Higouménaki's sign) is shown in a photograph that also depicts periostitis of the ribs. A beautiful photomicrograph of Wimberger's sign also has been included; this sign, which may appear in an infant with congenital syphilis, reveals radiolucency due to erosion of the medial aspect of the proximal tibial metaphysis.

The *Atlas* also includes a beautiful set of photographs which delineate the ophthalmologic examination of the newborn. Lesions which may result from trauma, infection, or congenital abnormalities are included. There are numerous photographs of the ocular manifestations of a variety of systemic diseases, such as Tay-Sachs disease, tuberous sclerosis, tyrosinase deficiency, and many more. Photographs of disturbances of each of the various organ systems, or disorders affecting such organ systems, also are included along with numerous photographs of different forms of dwarfism, nonchromosomal syndromes and associations, and chromosomal disorders. In short, this *Atlas* is the complete visual textbook of neonatology and will provide any physician, nurse, or student with a distillation of 50 years of neonatal experience as viewed through the eyes of a master clinician.

Arnold Jack Rudolph was born in 1918, grew up in South Africa, and graduated from the Witwatersrand Medical School in 1940. Following residency training in pediatrics at the Transvaal Memorial Hospital for Children, he entered private pediatric practice in Johannesburg, South Africa. After almost a decade, he left South Africa and moved to Boston, where he served as a Senior Assistant Resident in Medicine at the Children's Medical Center in Boston, Massachusetts, and subsequently pursued fellowship training in neonatology at the same institution and at the Boston Lying-In Hospital, Children's Medical Center and Harvard Medical School under Dr. Clement A. Smith.

In 1961, Dr. Rudolph came to Baylor College of Medicine in Houston, Texas, the school at which he spent the remainder of his career. He was a master teacher, who received the outstanding teacher award from pediatric medical students on so many occasions that he was elected to the Outstanding Faculty Hall of Fame in 1982. Dr. Rudolph also received numerous awards over the years from the pediatric house staffs for his superb teaching skills.

He was the Director of the Newborn Section in the Department of Pediatrics at Baylor College of Medicine for many years, until he voluntarily relinquished that position in 1986 for reasons related to his health.

Nevertheless, Jack Rudolph continued to work extraordinarily long hours in the care of the newborn infant, and was at the bedside teaching both students and house staff, as well as his colleagues, on a daily basis until just a few months before his death in July 1995.

Although Dr. Rudolph was the author or co-author of more than 100 published papers that appeared in the peer-reviewed medical literature, his most lasting contribution to neonatology and to pediatrics is in the legacy of the numerous medical students, house staff, fellows, and other colleagues whom he taught incessantly about how much one could learn from simply observing the newborn infant. This *Atlas* is a tour de force; it is a spectacular teaching tool that has been developed, collated, and presented by one of the finest clinical neonatologists in the history of medicine. It is an intensely personal volume that, as Dr. Rudolph himself states, "is not intended to rival standard neonatology texts," but rather to supplement them. This statement reveals Dr. Rudolph's innate modesty, since with the exception of some discussion on pathogenesis and treatment, it surpasses most neonatology texts in the wealth of clinical information that one can derive from viewing and imbibing its contents. We owe Dr. Rudolph and those who aided him in this work a debt of gratitude for making available to the medical community an unparalleled visual reference on the normal and abnormal newborn infant.

Ralph D. Feigin, M.D.
June 13, 1996

Preface

I first became attracted to the idea of producing a color atlas of neonatology many years ago. However, the impetus to synthesize my experience and compile this current collection was inspired by the frequent requests from medical students, pediatric house staff, nurses and others to provide them with a color atlas of the clinical material provided in my "slide shows." For the past few decades I have used the medium of color slides and radiographs as a teaching tool. In these weekly "slide shows" the normal and abnormal, as words never can, are illustrated.

"I cannot define an elephant but I know one when I see one."[1]

The collection of material used has been added to constantly with the support of the pediatric house staff who inform me to "bring your camera" whenever they see an unusual clinical finding or syndrome in the nurseries.

A thorough routine neonatal examination is the inalienable right of every infant. Most newborn babies are healthy and only a relatively small number may require special care. It is important to have the ability to distinguish normal variations and minor findings from the subtle early signs of problems. The theme that recurs most often is that careful clinical assessment, in the traditional sense, is the prerequisite and the essential foundation for understanding the disorders of the newborn. It requires familiarity with the wide range of normal, as well as dermatologic, cardiac, pulmonary, gastrointestinal, genitourinary, neurologic, and musculoskeletal disorders, genetics and syndromes. A background in general pediatrics and a working knowledge of obstetrics are essential. The general layout of the atlas is based on the above. Diseases are assigned to each section on the basis of the most frequent and obvious presenting sign. It seems probable that the findings depicted will change significantly in the decades to come. In this way duplication has been kept to a minimum. Additional space has been devoted to those areas of neonatal pathology (e.g., examination of the placenta, multiple births and iatrogenesis) which pose particular problems or cause clinical concern.

Obviously, because of limitations of space, it is impossible to be comprehensive and include every rare disorder or syndrome. I have tried to select both typical findings and variations in normal infants and those found in uncommon conditions. Some relevant conditions where individual variations need to be demonstrated are shown in more than one case.

As the present volume is essentially one of my personal experience, it is not intended to rival standard neonatology texts, but is presented as a supplement to them. It seems logical that references should be to standard texts or reviews where discussion on pathogenesis, treatment, and references to original works may be found.

Helen Mintz Hittner, M.D., has been kind enough to contribute the outstanding section on neonatal ophthalmology.

I have done my best to make the necessary acknowledgements to the various sources for the clinical material. If I have inadvertently omitted any of those, I apologize. My most sincere appreciation and thanks to Donna Hamburg, M.D., Kru Ferry, M.D., Michael Gomez, M.D., Virginia Schneider, PA, and Jeff Murray, M.D., who have spent innumerable hours in organizing and culling the material from my large collection. We wish to thank Abraham M. Rudolph, M.D., for his assistance in reviewing the material. We also wish to thank the following people for their photo contributions to this work: Cirilo Sotelo-Avila, Stan Connor, Avory Fanaroff, Milton Finegold, Brian Kershan, Tom Klima, Susan Landers, Gerardo Cabera-Meza, Ken Moise, Don Singer, Edward Singleton.

It is hoped that this atlas will provide neonatologists, pediatricians, family physicians, medical students and nurses with a basis for recognizing a broad spectrum of normal variations and clinical problems as well as provide them with an overall perspective of neonatology, a field in which there continues to be a rapid acceleration of knowledge and technology. One must bear in mind the caveat that pictures cannot supplant clinical experience in mastering the skill of visual recall.

1. Senile dementia of Alzheimer's type — normal aging or disease? (Editorial) *Lancet* 1989; i:476-477.

Arnold J. Rudolph, M.D.

CONTENTS

Volume II
Musculoskeletal Disorders and Congenital Deformities

Introduction

Although several texts provide extensive written descriptions of disorders of the newborn infant, the senses of touch, hearing and, especially, sight, create the most lasting impressions. Over a period of almost five decades, my brother Jack Rudolph diligently recorded in pictorial form his vast experiences in physical examination of the newborn infant. The *Atlas of the Newborn* reflects his selection from the thousands of color slides in his collection, and it truly represents the "art of medicine" as applied to neonatology. A number of unusual or rare conditions are included in this atlas. I consider this fully justified because, if one has not seen or heard of a condition, one cannot diagnose it.

This, the second of the five-volume series, includes three main topics: skeletal disorders, as well as dwarfism; multiple congenital anomaly syndromes; and chromosomal disorders.

Genetic skeletal disorders include a large group of anomalies which may be associated with dwarfism of various types, and may result in forcal structural or functional disorders. The examples of these disorders shorn in this volume draws attention to their appearance in the neonate, thus permitting early recognition of these anomalies.

Patients with multiple congenital anomaly syndromes and chromosomal disorders present a real challenge to the clinician, and recognition is often particularly difficult in the neonatal period. Although many descriptions of the various syndromes have been published, few provide good graphic examples. It is of utmost importance that these multiple congenital anomaly syndromes and chromosomal disorders be recognized as early as possible, so that appropriate therapeutic options, prognosis and recurrence risks can be presented to the families. The high quality photographs of various manifestations to these disorders will be of tremendous assistance to the clinician in recognizing them in the neonatal period.

This volume will be extremely valuable, not only to obstetricians, neonatologists and nurses involved in the perinatal period, but also to orthopaedists and clinical geneticists.

Abraham M. Rudolph, M.D.

Chapter 1
Musculoskeletal Disorders

Although some congenital musculoskeletal dysplasias are among the most obvious disorders of the neonate, they are also the most unusual. Congenital absence of all or part of a limb, deformities of the feet or hands, and lesions of the neck and trunk are rarely a diagnostic problem. The most common musculoskeletal dysplasias are among the most difficult to diagnose. Congenital hip dislocation may not be diagnosed even after repeated examination by experienced observers. Musculoskeletal infections complicating sepsis produce few subtle signs and may be easily overlooked. This is further complicated by the general concept that early diagnosis and treatment results in the greatest potential for normal growth and development of the infant. The examination of the musculoskeletal system should include inspection (e.g., looking for anomalies in contour position, and in spontaneous and reflex movement) and palpation (e.g., to determine if there are abnormalities in passive motion) and should be systematic to ensure completeness.

1.1

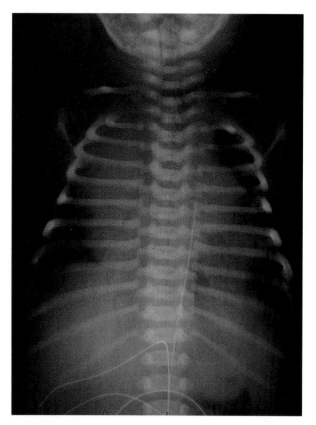

Figure 1.1. Chest radiograph showing 11 ribs. The presence of 11 ribs is not an uncommon finding in normal infants but occurs with greater frequency in infants with Down syndrome. Note the cardiac enlargement and enlarged thymus.

1.2

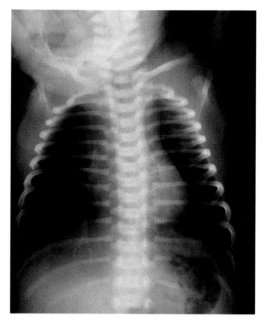

Figure 1.2. Radiograph showing 13 ribs bilaterally in an otherwise normal infant.

1.3

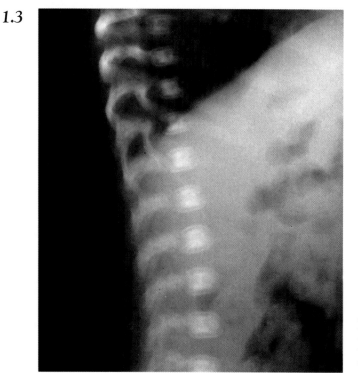

Figure 1.3. Lateral radiograph of the spine showing the "bone-in-bone" appearance of the vertebral bodies. This is a striking example of growth arrest but otherwise is a nonspecific finding.

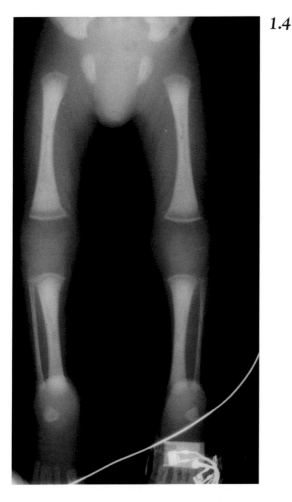

1.4

Figure 1.4. This figure shows the growth arrest lines in the long bones of a term infant with severe intrauterine growth retardation. Note the lack of the distal femoral and proximal tibial ossification centers, normally appearing at 36 and 38 weeks respectively, also caused by growth retardation. Hypothyroidism is also a consideration.

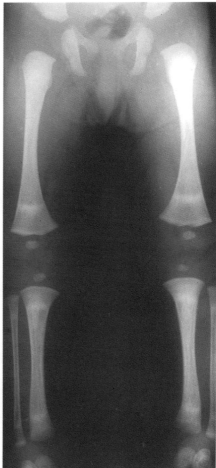

1.5

Figure 1.5. A radiograph of the lower extremities in a term infant showing the growth arrest lines. Note that in this infant the distal femoral tibial and proximal tibial ossification centers are present.

Figure 1.6. A radiograph showing faulty segmentation of vertebrae in an infant with rachischisis. This defect may be seen in infants with the VATER syndrome and other congenital anomalies.

Hemivertebrae may occur in the cervical or thoracic spine, and less commonly in the lumbar spine. An isolated hemivertebra may not be recognized clinically but can cause abnormal posture (scoliosis). More commonly, hemivertebrae are multiple and may be associated with other skeletal abnormalities, as in the ribs.

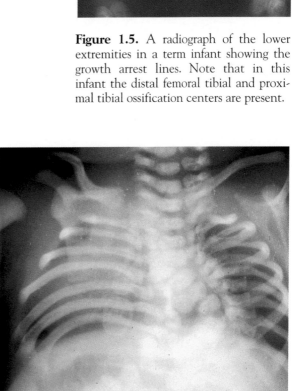

1.6

1.7

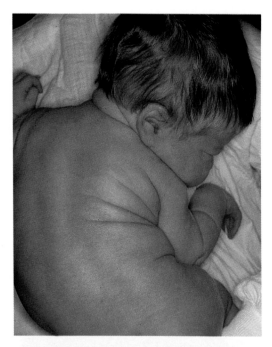

Figure 1.7. Congenital scoliosis is rare in neonates but may occur in association with structural anomalies of the vertebral spine. In this infant, the congenital scoliosis was associated with abnormal segmentation of vertebrae.

1.8

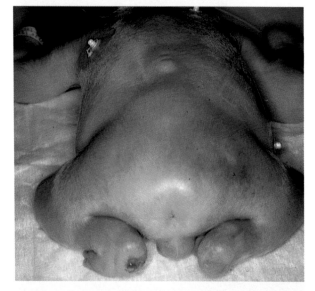

Figure 1.8. In this infant with caudal regression syndrome, the mother was a class B diabetic. Oligohydramnios was present, but renal function was normal in the infant. Note the arthrogryposis of the lower extremities.

1.9

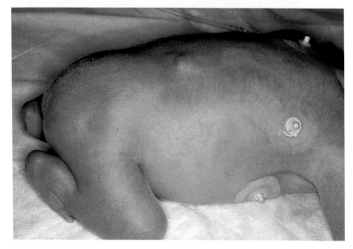

Figure 1.9. Lateral view of the same infant showing the prominent end of the spine and arthrogryposis of the lower extremities.

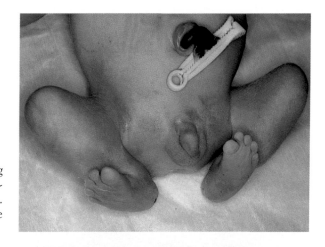

1.10

Figure 1.10. Frontal view of the same infant showing the short lower extremities due to the marked arthrogryposis affecting the hip, knee, and ankle joints. Infants with lumbosacral agenesis clinically adopt the so-called "Buddha" position.

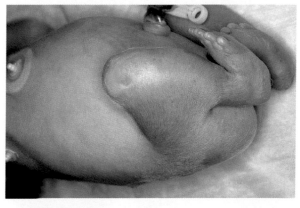

1.11

Figure 1.11. The same infant showing the arthrogryposis but note the dimple at the knee. Skin dimples such as this are associated with pressure over a joint and lack of movement.

1.12

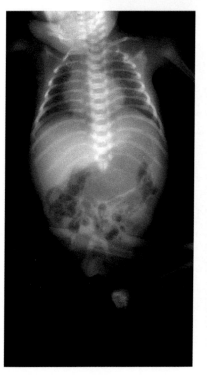
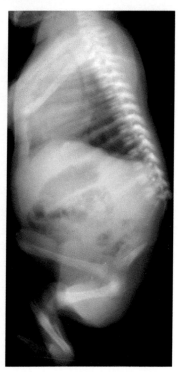

Figure 1.12. Anteroposterior and lateral radiographs demonstrating the lumbosacral agenesis.

1.13

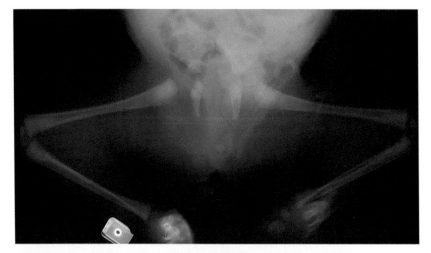

Figure 1.13. Radiograph of the lower extremities of the same infant. Note the abnormal development of the pelvis due to the lumbosacral agenesis, the thin, poorly developed bones and lack of muscle mass. This is due to lack of fetal movement and resulting arthrogryposis.

1.14

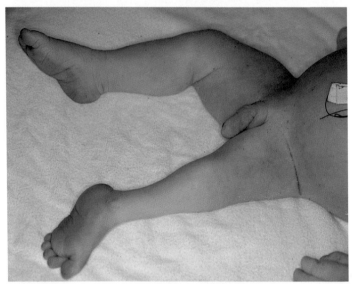

Figure 1.14. An asymmetric form of the caudal regression syndrome and hypoplastic left lower extremity associated with hypoplasia of muscles and sciatic nerve on the left side.

1.15

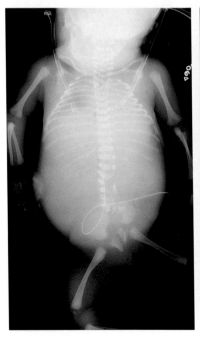
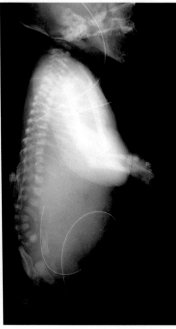

Figure 1.15. Anteroposterior and lateral radiographs of the same infant. Note the hemicaudal dysplasia. Also note the bilateral pulmonary hypoplasia.

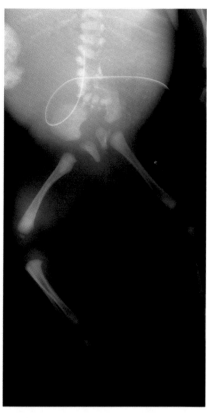

1.16

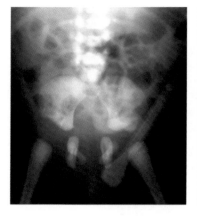

1.17

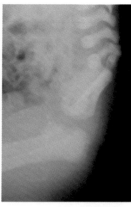

Figure 1.17. Anteroposterior and lateral radiograph of an infant with sacral agenesis, born to a diabetic mother. This is one of the classic abnormalities reported in infants of diabetic mothers.

Figure 1.16. Close-up radiograph of the pelvis and lower extremities in the same infant. There are lumbar and sacral hemivertebrae with left scoliosis and vertebral fusion, hypoplasia of left pelvic bones, dislocation of the left hip, and a hypoplastic left lower extremity.

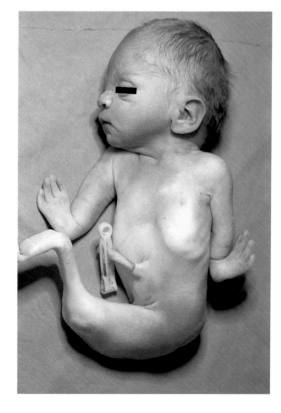

1.18

Figure 1.18. Sirenomelia ("mermaid" fetus) in an infant of a diabetic mother shows the severe postural deformities associated with the oligohydramnios which is always present in infants with sirenomelia because of renal agenesis. These infants typically lack an anus and have abnormal genitalia. Note the Potter facies, low-set ears, epicanthal folds and micrognathia associated with oligohydramnios and renal agenesis.

1.19

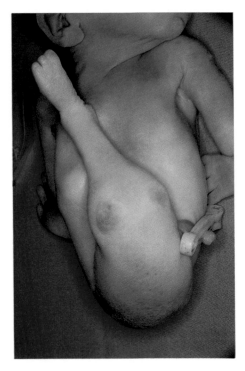

Figure 1.19. The same infant as in Fig. 1.18 placed in its position-of-comfort in utero. Note that the fused lower extremities give the typical appearance of a mermaid.

1.20

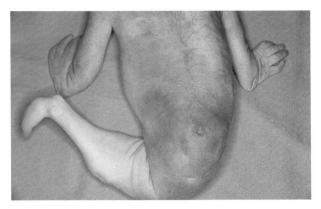

Figure 1.20. Note the anal atresia and postural deformities of the hands and lower body in the same infant.

1.21

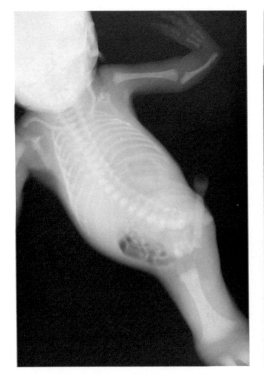

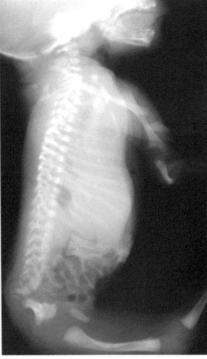

Figure 1.21. Anteroposterior and lateral radiographs of the same infant show the marked scoliosis, the abnormal pelvis and the fused femora.

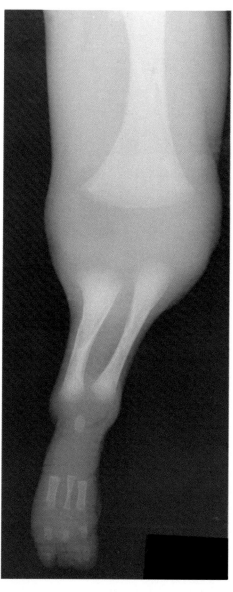

1.22

Figure 1.22. Radiograph of the same infant showing the fused femora, separate tibiae and abnormal development of the foot.

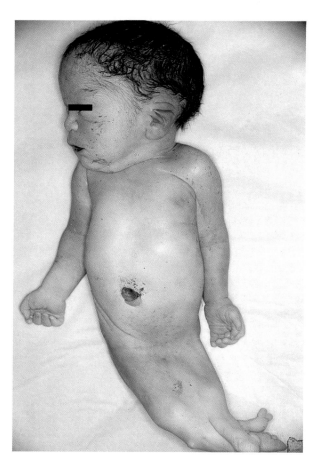

1.23

Figure 1.23. This infant of a diabetic mother exhibits sirenomelia with total lack of development of the genitalia and an imperforate anus. Associated with the renal agenesis is oligohydramnios; this infant also demonstrates the typical Potter facies. Note the low-set ear, flat nose and micrognathia.

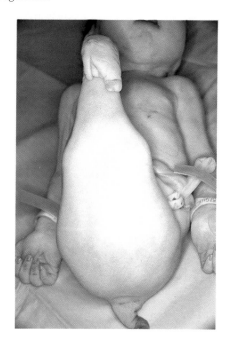

1.24

Figure 1.24. Sirenomelia in another infant of a diabetic mother; the infant had severe oligohydramnios associated with renal agenesis. There were no external genitalia and anal atresia was present, but note that this infant had a "tail" present.

1.25

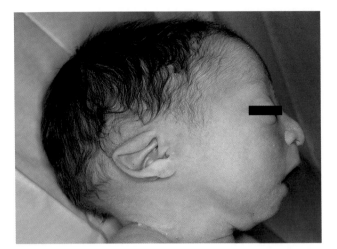

Figure 1.25. A close-up of the face of the same infant with the typical Potter facies associated with oligohydramnios and renal agenesis. Note the low-set abnormal ears, the flat nose, and micrognathia. Epicanthal folds were also present.

1.26

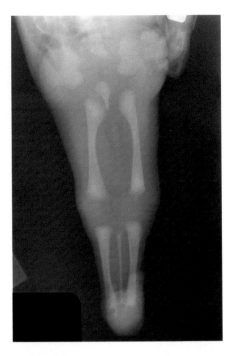

Figure 1.26. Radiograph of the lower extremities of the same infant with sirenomelia shows the presence of two separate femora with fusion of soft tissue, two separate tibiae, and a single fibula distally.

SKELETAL DEFICIENCIES

Skeletal deficiencies may be longitudinal defects which affect the limb on one side of the central axis or transverse defects in which the limb is truncated abruptly and the limb may terminate at any level but distal involvement is more common than proximal. Thus, radial aplasia with absence of the thumb and forefinger is characterized as a preaxial longitudinal hemimelia of the upper limb. Similarly, involvement of the lower limb would produce tibial aplasia. The affected limb will be curved toward the side of the deficiency and usually will be somewhat foreshortened. In transverse defects the defect closely resembles a congenital amputation but usually there is some degree of hypoplasia of the remaining proximal structures and the distal stump of the limb is not scarred but commonly small nubbins of tissue representing rudimentary digits may be present. Differentiation should be made between transverse defects, which are primary limb reduction defects, and secondary limb reduction defects which arise as a result of disruption.

1.27

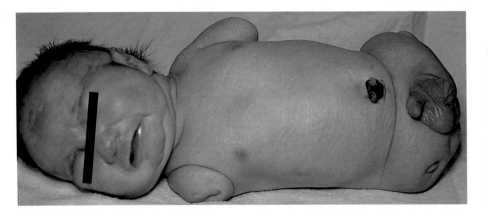

Figure 1.27. Amelia of all extremities (tetramelia). Amelia is absence of the entire limb structure. There was a history of consanguinity. Apart from the abnormalities of the extremities, this infant was normal.

1.28

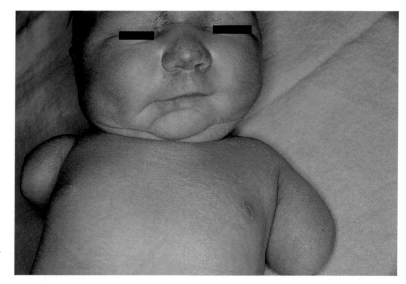

Figure 1.28. Close-up of the upper extremities of the same infant.

1.29

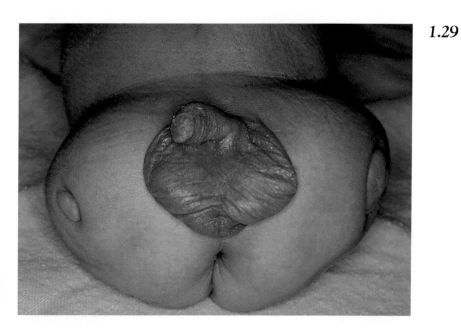

Figure 1.29. Close-up of the lower extremities of the same infant.

1.30

Figure 1.30. An infant with amelia of the upper extremities and ectromelia of the lower extremities. Ectromelia is the absence or incomplete development of the long bones of one or more of the limbs. This may represent the most extreme form of an intercalary defect. In total amelia, a form of ectromelia, no limb elements whatsoever are present.

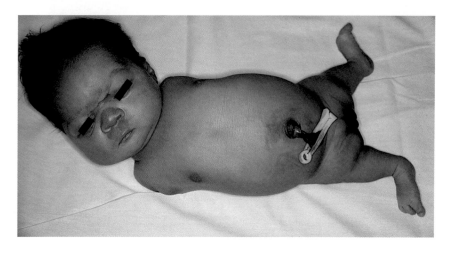

1.31

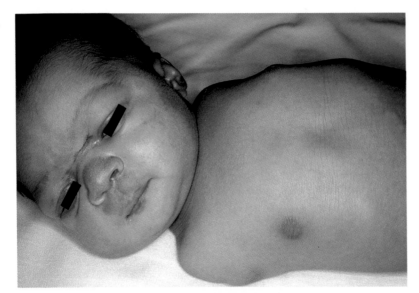

Figure 1.31. Close-up of amelia of upper extremities of the same infant. This infant had abnormal scapulae.

1.32

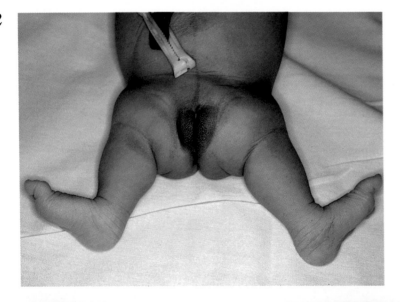

Figure 1.32. Close-up of ectromelia of the lower extremities of the same infant.

1.33

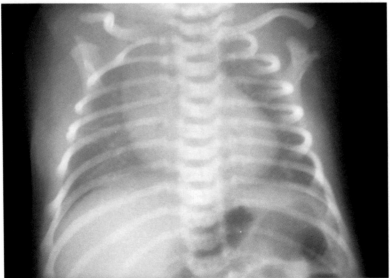

Figure 1.33. Chest radiograph of the same infant. Note the abnormal scapulae and total absence of the upper extremities. This radiograph stresses the importance of looking at the total radiograph and not the lungs alone when looking at a chest radiograph.

Figure 1.34. In a radiograph of the lower extremities of the same infant, note that there are no hip joints and that the femora and fibulae are absent bilaterally.

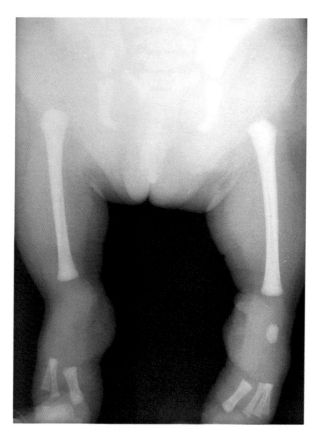

1.34

INTERCALARY DEFECTS

Intercalary defects are those in which a more proximal portion of a limb fails to develop properly but distal structures are relatively intact. An extreme example is phocomelia, which involves partial or complete underdevelopment of the rhizomelic and mesomelic limb segments. The structures of the hands and feet may be reduced to a single digit or may appear relatively normal but arise directly from the trunk like the flippers of a seal. In less severe cases, portions of the proximal limb may remain.

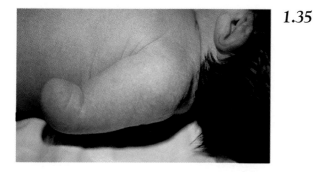

1.35

Figure 1.35. This otherwise normal infant has an isolated limb malformation of the left arm. This is a transverse defect and is a primary limb reduction defect.

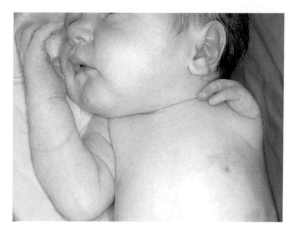

1.36

Figure 1.36. This infant represents an example of unilateral non-thalidomide-induced phocomelia. This malformation, which was common in thalidomide-exposed babies, is, otherwise, a very rare congenital malformation.

1.37

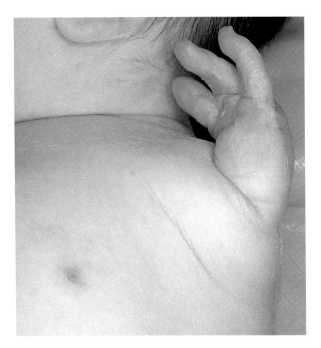

1.38

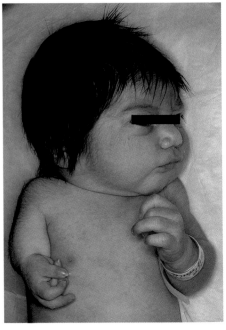

Figure 1.37. Close-up of the phocomelia in the same infant as in Figure 1.36. This is a primary limb reduction defect in that there was lack of the humerus, radius, and ulna in the left upper extremity. In phocomelia there may be absence of the femur, tibia, and fibula in the lower extremities. There may be bilateral involvement of the extremities.

Figure 1.38. Hemimelia of the right upper extremity. This is another example of a transverse defect in which a limb is truncated abruptly. This is a primary limb reduction defect.

1.39

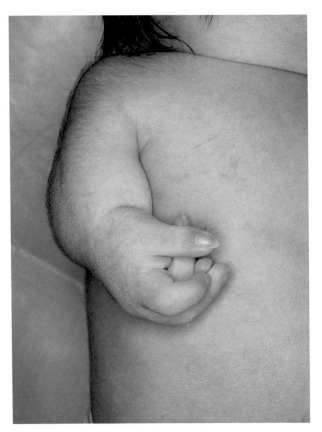

Figure 1.39. Close-up of hemimelia in same infant. Note the well-developed hand.

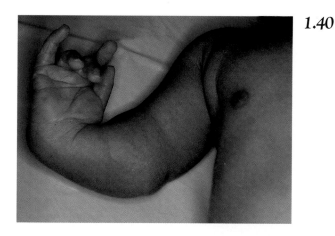

1.40

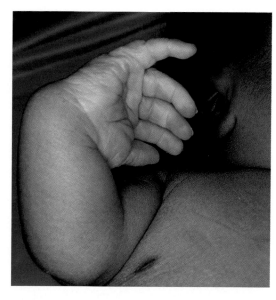

1.41

Figure 1.40. This infant has the thrombocytopenia-absent radius (TAR) syndrome. There is absence of the radius bilaterally. Note that the absence of the radius of the right forearm has resulted in a "club hand." In the TAR syndrome the thumb is always present.

Clinical signs of radial dysplasia include a shortening of the forearm with radial displacement of the hand ("club hand"). Varying degrees of dysplasia occur, ranging from complete absence of the radius with major malformations of the preaxial (radial) side of the hand to normal development of the radius and only minor anomalies of the thumb.

Figure 1.41. Another view of the same infant with the TAR syndrome showing the left forearm and hand. Again note the presence of the thumb. Some dysmorphic syndromes, such as the TAR syndrome, may show varying combinations of the different types of limb defect. There is a preaxial longitudinal defect (absence of the radius), but the ulna is also short and the thumb and forefinger are invariably present as expected with an intercalary defect.

Radial dysplasia may be associated with pancytopenia as in Fanconi's syndrome but may also be associated with congenital heart disease and abnormalities of other parts of the skeleton.

Figure 1.42. This infant has Fanconi's syndrome. Note the congenital absence of the right radius and right thumb. In Fanconi's syndrome the thumb may occasionally be present. Note the club hand with absence of the radius and the thumb. This may be unilateral or bilateral. In Fanconi's syndrome there is pancytopenia (anemia, neutropenia, and thrombocytopenia) in addition to the hypoplastic or absent thumbs and hypoplastic or absent radius.

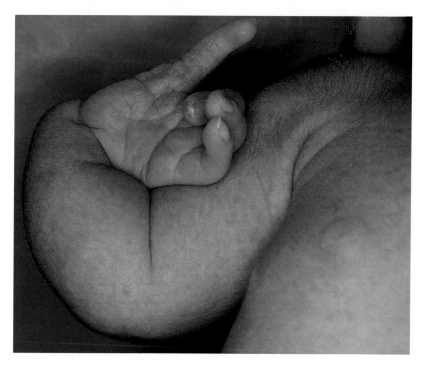

1.42

1.43

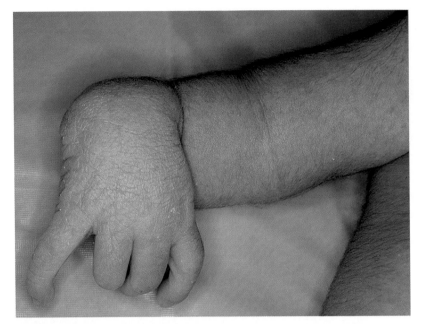

Figure 1.43. Another view of the same infant as in Figure 1.42 showing the absence of the radius and right thumb with the typical club hand.

1.44

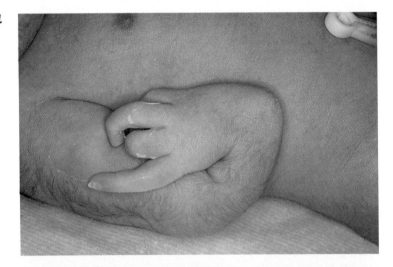

Figure 1.44. Another example of Fanconi's syndrome with congenital absence of the right radius and thumb and thrombocytopenia (platelet count of 30,000/mm^3). Note the skin dimples at the elbow which are related to the infant's position in utero.

1.45

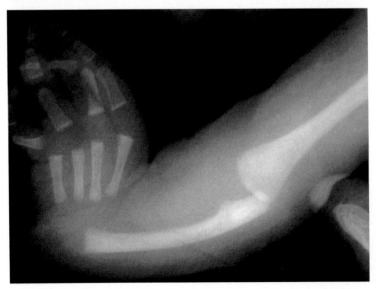

Figure 1.45. Radiograph of the right upper extremity of the same infant showing the absence of the radius and right thumb.

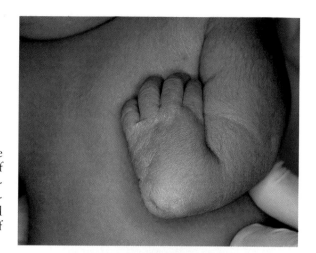

1.46

Figure 1.46. In this infant with Holt-Oram syndrome (cardiac limb syndrome), note the congenital absence of the left radius and thumb. The infant also had coarctation of the aorta. Holt-Oram syndrome may be associated with any congenital cardiac defect of which atrial septal defect is the most common. A family history of this condition is common.

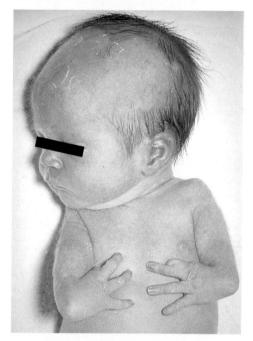

1.47

Figure 1.47. Bilateral congenital absence of thumbs and radii in an otherwise normal infant. The father of this infant had the same congenital abnormalities. It is important to obtain a good family history as this condition may be familial.

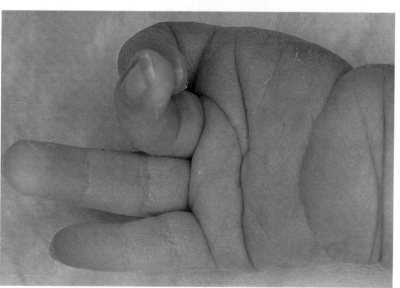

1.48

Figure 1.48. Congenital absence of the right thumb was present in this otherwise normal infant.

1.49

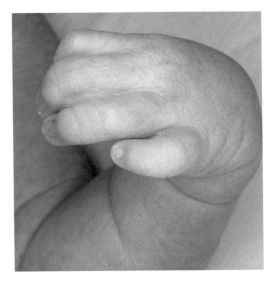

Figure 1.49. Another example of congenital absence of the thumb in an otherwise normal infant but note there is syndactyly between the third and fourth fingers.

1.50

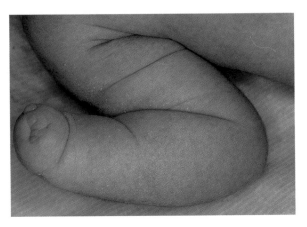

Figure 1.50. Acheiria of the right hand in an infant. This occurs because of a failure of formation of the hand as an isolated defect. The radius and ulna may be foreshortened, there are no metacarpals or phalanges seen radiologically, the thumb may be normally formed, and rudimentary nails may be present. This is an example of a transverse defect in which there is hypoplasia of all structures distal to a particular level on the limb. Usually there is preservation of the more proximal parts which may be normal or diminished in size.

1.51

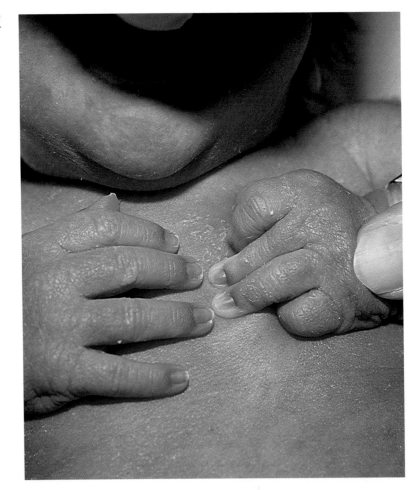

Figure 1.51. This otherwise normal infant had microcheiria of the left hand. Note the normal right hand. The normal hand is about twice as long as it is wide. If metacarpal hypoplasia is present it produces an unusually short palm.

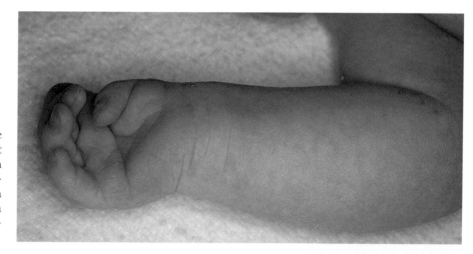

1.52

Figure 1.52. Note the microcheiria of the right hand in this infant with Cornelia de Lange's syndrome. This is not an uncommon finding in infants with this syndrome.

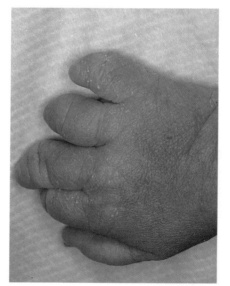
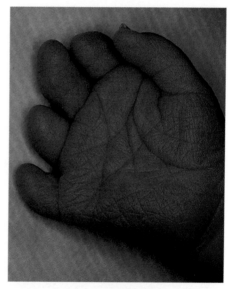

1.53

Figure 1.53. Brachydactyly of the right hand. This finding may be isolated but is seen in many syndromes.

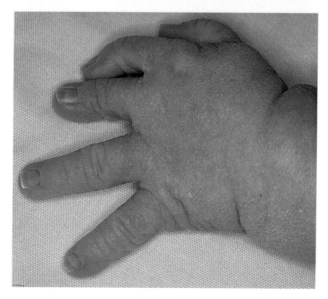

1.54

Figure 1.54. Dorsal view of congenital brachydactyly of the index and middle fingers of left hand. The father had the identical type of congenital brachydactyly.

Asymmetric length of the fingers is usually the result of hypoplasia of one or more phalanges. Tapered fingers may indicate mild hypoplasia of the middle and distal phalanges.

1.55

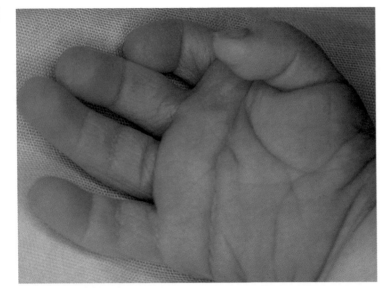

Figure 1.55. Ventral view of the right hand of the same infant as in Figure 1.54.

1.56

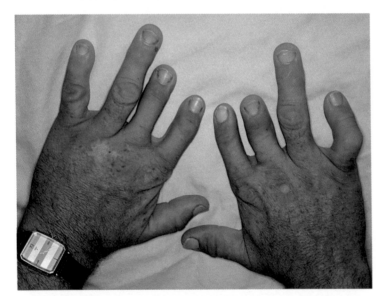

Figure 1.56. Identical bilateral congenital brachydactyly in the infant's father.

1.57

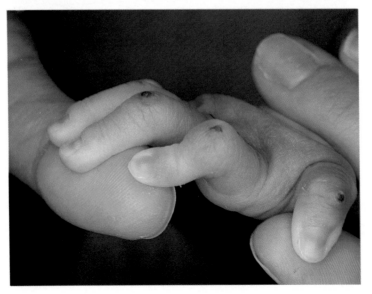

Figure 1.57. Camptodactyly (bent, contracted digits) most commonly affects the fifth, fourth and third digits in decreasing order of frequency. Presumably, it is the consequence of relative shortness in the length of the flexor tendons with respect to growth of the hand. It may occur as an isolated finding but is more commonly associated with lack of movement in utero. It is usually bilateral and symmetrical. Each finger should be extended passively to its full extent. Extension of less than 180 degrees at any joint signifies joint contracture (camptodactyly).

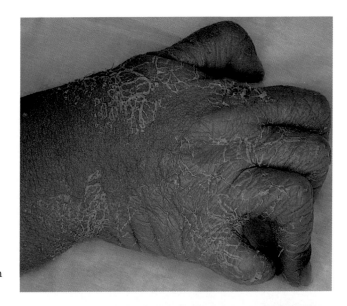

1.58

Figure 1.58. Camptodactyly of fingers in an infant with arthrogryposis.

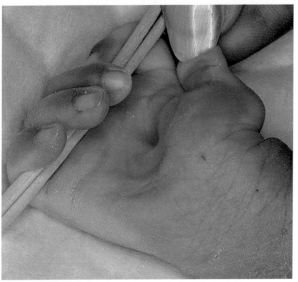

1.59

Figure 1.59. The hand of the same infant showing the severity of the contractures and lack of palmar creases due to the severe contractures. Note the depression in the palm resulting from the contracted fingers.

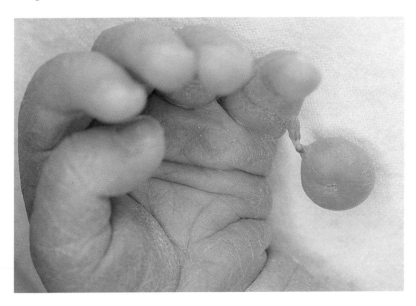

1.60

Figure 1.60. Supernumerary digit in which the thin pedicle distinguishes it from true polydactyly. In polydactyly the additional digit may consist solely of soft tissue or less commonly has skeletal elements.

1.61

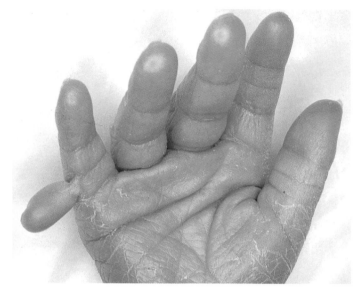

Figure 1.61. Postaxial polydactyly is most commonly seen in black infants where it occurs as an autosomal dominant trait. The polydactyly may be noted as a nubbin of scar tissue, as a pedunculated mass attached by a small pedicle, or as a fully developed digit. Polydactyly may be preaxial, occurring at the thumb or big toe, or postaxial, arising on the ulnar aspect of the fifth finger or fibular aspect of the fifth toe. Central polydactyly does occur but is extremely rare. The vast majority of infants with polydactyly have postaxial polydactyly.

1.62

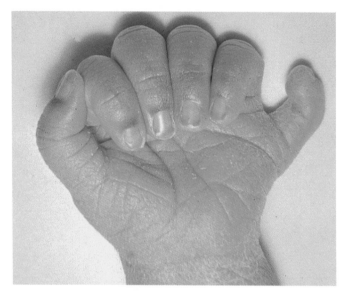

Figure 1.62. Another example of postaxial polydactyly with a well-developed digit. These digits may be fairly well formed with one or more rudimentary phalanges. Duplication of digits occurs when one or more extra digital rays are formed during the embryonic period. Polydactyly is an associated finding in many syndromes such as trisomy 13 or 18, Ellis-van Creveld syndrome, Carpenter's syndrome, etc.

1.63

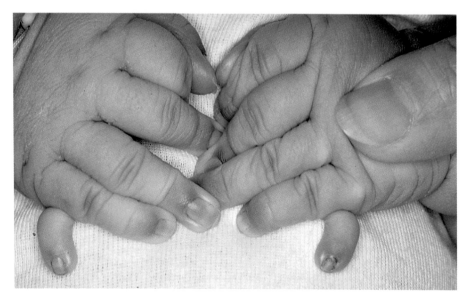

Figure 1.63. Bilateral postaxial polydactyly. Note that polydactyly may be unilateral or bilateral.

1.64

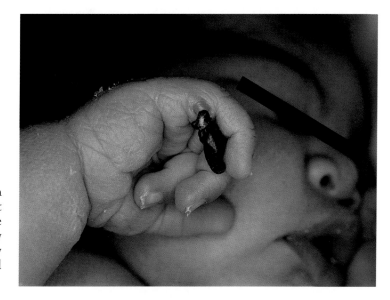

Figure 1.64. Postaxial polydactyly in an infant at birth showing a necrotic, almost amputated, extra digit due to interference with circulation. This would explain why some infants with polydactyly may only have evidence of scarring on the lateral side of the digit.

1.65

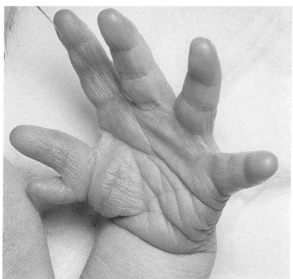

Figure 1.65. This infant has preaxial polydactyly of the right hand. Preaxial polydactyly is less common but has the same range of severity, with the accessory tissue usually arising from the midportion of the thumb or first toe.

1.66

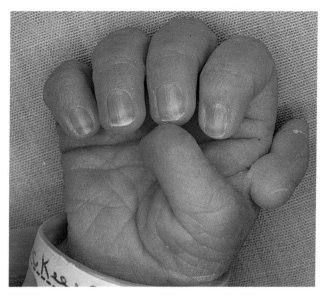

Figure 1.66. In this infant with preaxial polydactyly, note that the extra digit is poorly developed.

1.67

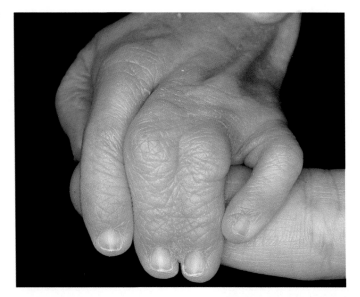

Figure 1.67. Partial cutaneous syndactyly represents an incomplete separation of the fingers and occurs most commonly between the third and fourth fingers and between the second and third toes. Syndactyly is the most frequent form of hand anomaly. It is often bilateral and may be combined with polydactyly, congenital finger amputations, and syndromes. Syndactyly refers to fusion of the soft tissues without synostosis (bony fusion). If there is synostosis, the term symphalangism is used.

1.68

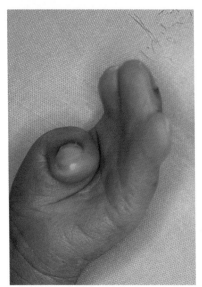 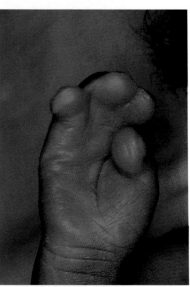

Figure 1.68. This infant with Apert's syndrome (acrocephalosyndactyly) shows symmetric syndactyly of both hands. In Apert's syndrome, total syndactyly may involve the full length of the hands or feet. They appear cupped and mitten-like and may have a single undulating band-shaped nail.

1.69

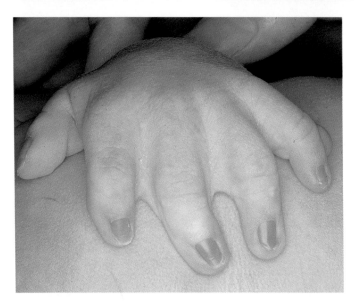

Figure 1.69. In Carpenter's syndrome (acrocephalopolysyndactyly), polysyndactyly is a prominent feature. Note the webbing between the digits; the extra digit can be noted behind the fifth digit.

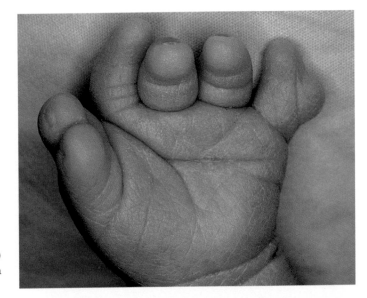

Figure 1.70. Polysyndactyly (seven digits) with brachydactyly and hypoplastic nails in an infant with Ellis-van Creveld syndrome.

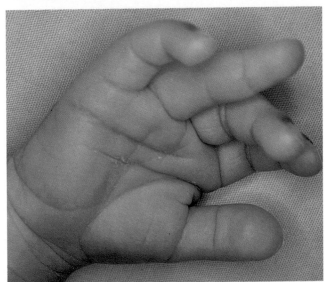

Figure 1.71. There was a family history of broad thumbs and toes in this otherwise normal infant who exhibits an overgrowth anomaly of the thumbs and big toes. Syndromes such as Rubenstein-Taybi and Larsen's syndrome should be excluded in infants with broad thumbs and toes.

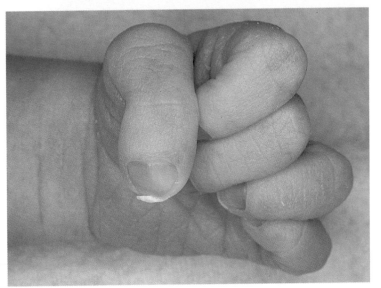

Figure 1.72. A broad spatulate thumb in an infant with Larsen's syndrome.

1.73

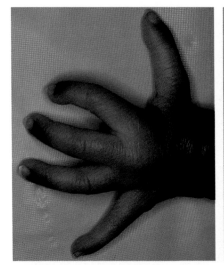 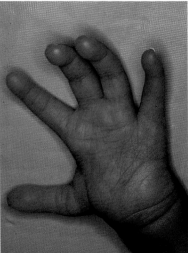

Figure 1.73. A dorsal (left) and ventral (right) view of digitalization of the right thumb in an infant with imperforate anus and microphthalmia. Karyotype was normal.

If there are three phalanges comprising the thumb (triphalangeal thumb), conditions such as Fanconi's pancytopenia syndrome and Holt-Oram syndrome should be considered in the differential diagnosis. A triphalangeal thumb lies in the same plane as the fingers.

1.74

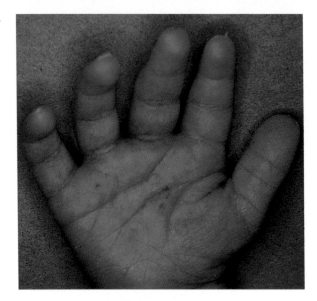

Figure 1.74. A palmar view of digitalization of the right thumb in another infant. Note the extra creases in the thumb. This infant also had bifid big toes with polydactyly.

1.75

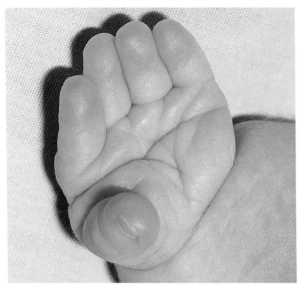

Figure 1.75. The "hitchhiker" thumb is a proximally placed thumb caused by hypoplasia of the first metacarpal. The thumb is retroflexed with hypoplasia of the thenar eminence. This type of thumb is typical in diastrophic dwarfism.

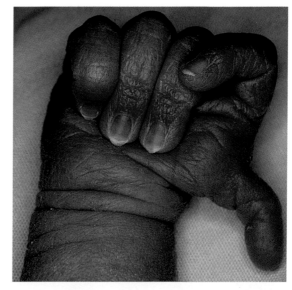

Figure 1.76. Pouce flottant ("floating" thumb) of the right hand. In this condition there is an absent or hypoplastic first metacarpal.

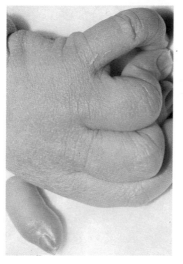

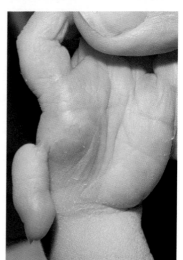

Figure 1.77. Another example of pouce flottant. There is an absence or maldevelopment of the first metacarpal with phalanges.

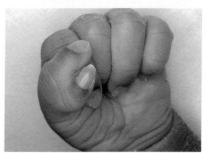

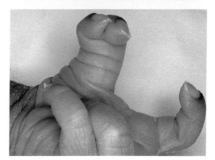

Figure 1.78. An early insult to the limb bud in the 5th to 6th embryologic week may result in a duplication of parts, especially of the hands and feet, such as this bifid thumb.

1.79

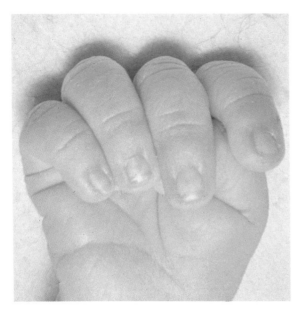

Figure 1.79. Palmar adduction ("cortical" thumb) in a normal infant. The thumbs are freely mobile but are held adducted and flexed across the palms with the fingers tightly clutched over them. "Cortical" thumbs are a manifestation of hypertonicity when they are present beyond the first 3 to 4 months. Constant palmar adduction or "clasped" thumb after this age would alert one to the possibility of central nervous system pathology. "Clasped" thumbs are held in a flexed and adducted position across the palm and cannot be abducted or extended.

1.80

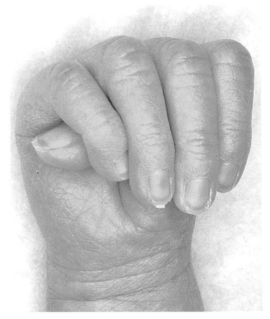

Figure 1.80. In infants with neonatal Marfan syndrome, the thumb may extend beyond the fifth finger when the infant fists its hand. This infant with Marfan syndrome had an upper/lower segment ratio of 1.52. The normal upper/lower segment ratio in the neonate is 1.69 to 1.7. It is much reduced in Marfan syndrome and increased in short-limbed dwarfism and hypothyroidism. Note that the fingers are long, tubular, and relatively slender.

1.81

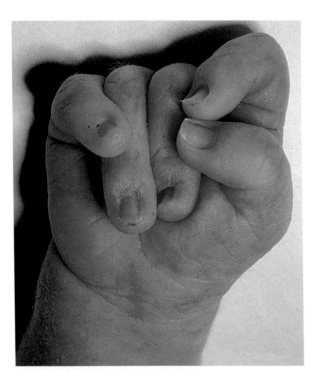

Figure 1.81. The typical appearance of the fingers in trisomy 18. Note the index finger overlapping the third finger and the fifth finger overlapping the fourth finger. Also note the hypoplastic nails.

1.82

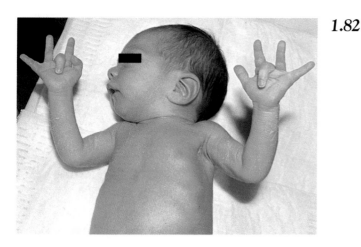

1.83

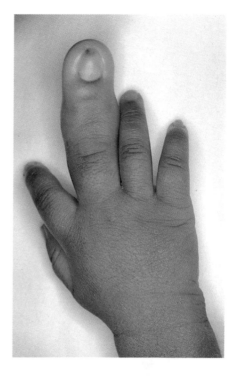

Figure 1.82. Bilateral trigger fingers in a neonate. Trigger digits may involve the thumbs or the fingers. The fingers may present with clicking, flexion contractures of the proximal interphalangeal joint, or both. They are much less commonly involved than the thumbs which present with a palpable nodule at the proximal flexor tendon pulley at the level of the metacarpophalangeal joint. Trigger thumbs must be distinguished from a congenital clasped thumb in which the deformity usually affects the metacarpophalangeal joint.

Figure 1.83. Macrodactyly of the right middle finger occurring from a localized overgrowth of a digit. This occurs most frequently as a random isolated enlargement of a finger or toe, or it may be associated with vascular or lymphatic malformations or may occur in neurofibromatosis.

1.84

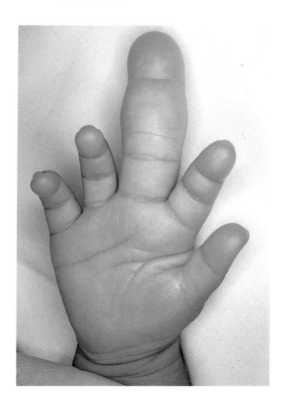

Figure 1.84. Ventral view of the macrodactyly of the right middle finger in the same infant. This was an isolated finding in this infant.

1.85

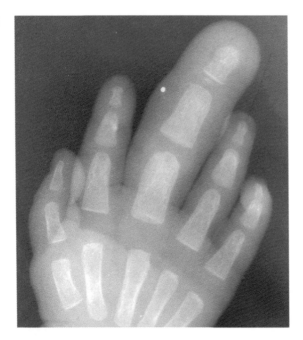

Figure 1.85. Radiograph of the hand of the infant shown in Figure 1.84 showing the macrodactyly of the right middle finger.

1.86

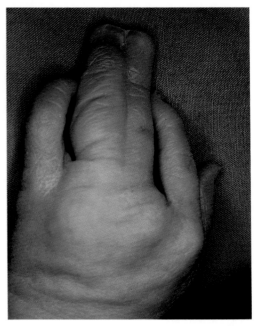

Figure 1.86. Macrosyndactyly of the third and fourth fingers of the left hand. This infant had a massive diffuse lymphangioma involving the left side of the neck, the chest, and the upper extremity.

1.87

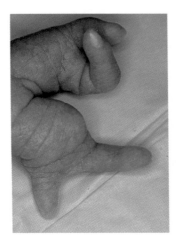 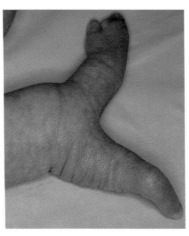

Figure 1.87. In these infants with "lobster-claw" deformity (ectrodactyly, or split hand/split foot deformation), the typical V-shaped cleft is noted on the left. In this classic form, all four limbs are involved. The feet are usually more severely affected than the hands. This type is strongly familial and is usually inherited as an autosomal dominant. The atypical type of lobster-claw deformity is seen on the right. Note that the cleft is wider (U-shaped defect) with only a thumb and small finger remaining. This atypical type has no genetic basis and usually involves a single upper extremity but always spares the feet.

1.88

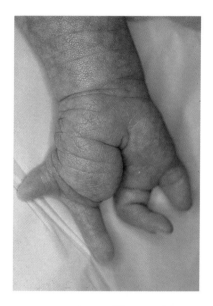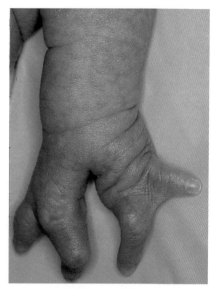

Figure 1.88. Typical V-shaped lobster-claw deformity of the hands. The lobster-claw deformity may be associated with other malformations, often as a genetically determined syndrome. In the hand, the typical deformity consists of the absence of the third digital ray, with a deep triangular cleft extending to the level of the carpal bones. Fingers bordering the cleft may show clinodactyly, camptodactyly, or syndactyly and are sometimes hypoplastic or completely missing.

1.89

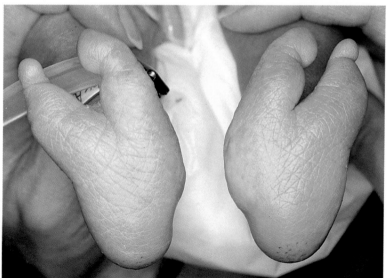

Figure 1.89. The typical V-shaped lobster-claw deformity of the feet in the same infant.

1.90

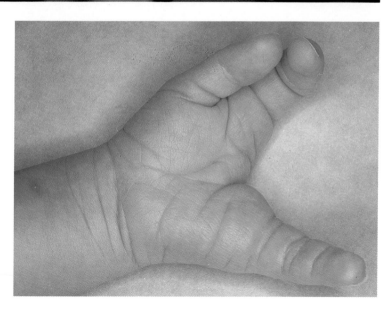

Figure 1.90. The atypical type of lobster-claw deformity (U-shaped defect) which only involved the right hand of this infant. Note the wider cleft. This is a sporadic defect.

1.91

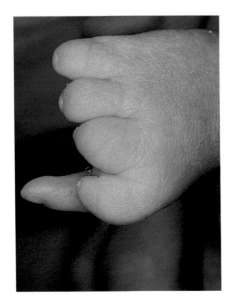

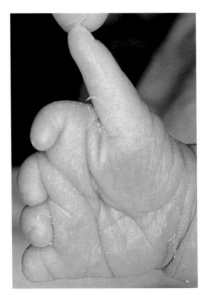

Figure 1.91. A primary reduction malformation of the fingers of the right hand.

1.92

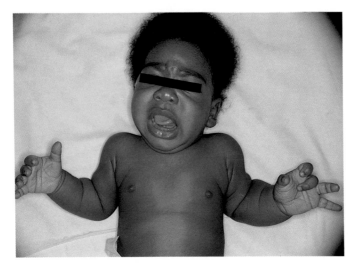

Figure 1.92. Congenital hypertrophy of the left upper extremity of an infant at the age of five months. This is also known as segmental hypertrophy or local acromegaly. This is often not obvious at birth but becomes more apparent with increasing age. Limb asymmetry can be caused by vascular anomalies that produce localized overcirculation, but more commonly is found as an isolated phenomenon. When such asymmetry affects one entire side of the body, the term hemihypertrophy is used.

Differential diagnosis of hemihypertrophy includes neurofibromatosis, Wilms' tumor, Beckwith-Wiedemann syndrome, Klippel-Trénaunay syndrome, and Russell-Silver dwarf, but most commonly this is an idiopathic finding.

1.93

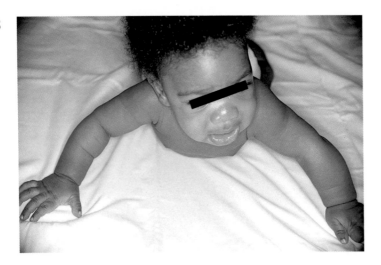

Figure 1.93. The same infant demonstrating the congenital hypertrophy of the left upper extremity.

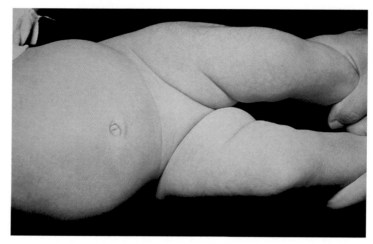

1.94

Figure 1.94. A frontal view of a neonate with congenital dislocation of the hip. Note the asymmetry of the skin folds. In congenital dislocation of the hip, asymmetry is not commonly noted in the neonatal period. Congenital dislocation is very much more common in female infants.

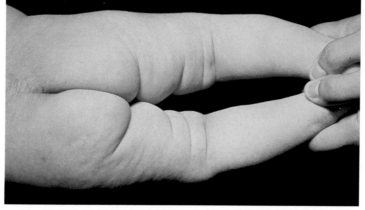

1.95

Figure 1.95. A dorsal view of the same infant shows the asymmetric gluteal folds and other skin folds. In the neonatal period the asymmetry of the gluteal folds and other skin folds is usually not as apparent as it is in this infant.

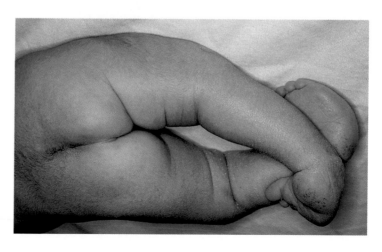

1.96

Figure 1.96. Congenital hip dislocation and bilateral club feet in an infant with Poland's anomaly. Note the asymmetry of the creases. Congenital hip dislocation is commonly associated with the presence of other congenital postural deformities. Also note the bilateral talipes equinovarus.

1.97

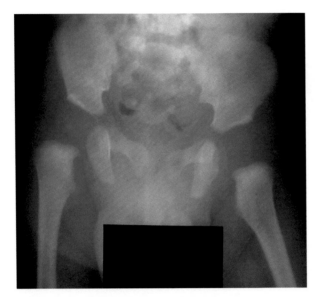

Figure 1.97. Radiograph of congenital dislocation of the hip.

1.98

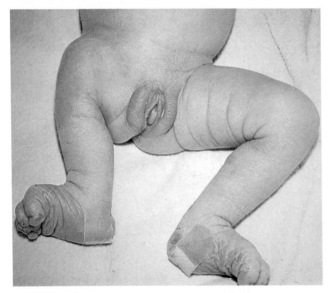

Figure 1.98. Proximal focal femoral deficiency of the right side in an otherwise normal infant. This is a congenital defect of unknown cause, usually consisting of a shortening and contracture of the proximal portion of the femur with or without involvement of the pelvic bones. The severity of the condition depends on the presence or absence of the femoral head and acetabulum. Treatment is directed towards stabilizing the hip. Correction of the leg length discrepancy may require an amputation above the knee and fitting with a prosthesis.

1.99

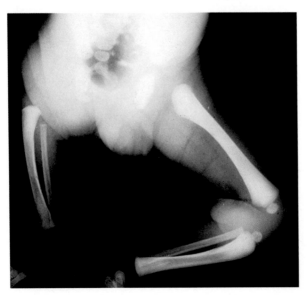

Figure 1.99. Radiograph of the same infant showing the proximal focal femoral deficiency.

1.100

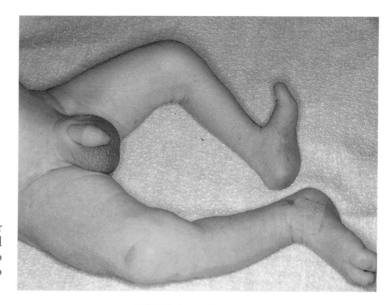

Figure 1.100. Hypotrophic left lower extremity. This may occur in the caudal regression syndrome or may be due to interference with the vascular supply to the lower extremity.

1.101

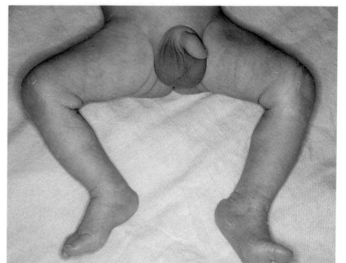

Figure 1.101. Hypoplastic right lower extremity with four toes on the right foot.

1.102

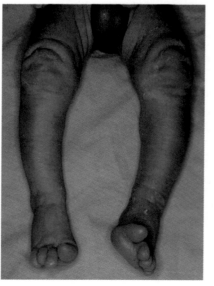
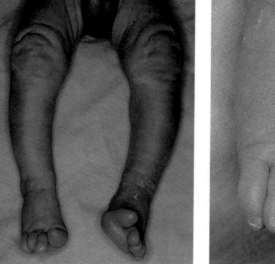

Figure 1.102. The same infant showing the hypoplasia of the right lower extremity and the presence of four toes on the right foot. Note that the hypoplasia can be subtle.

1.103

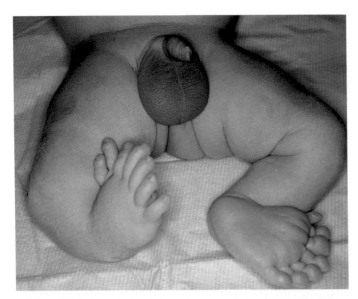

Figure 1.103. Congenital absence of patellae in a normal infant. This finding is also noted in trisomy 8 and Nievergelt syndrome.

1.104

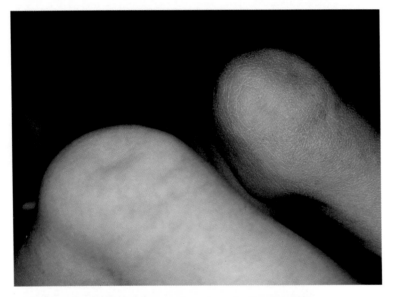

Figure 1.104. In this infant with the tibia reduction-polydactyly syndrome there is an absence of the tibiae bilaterally with septadactyly on the right foot and octadactyly on the left foot. Absence or hypoplasia of the tibia was seen in the thalidomide syndrome. It is otherwise rare, whereas absence of the fibula is more common. It is more common in males, more often unilateral and more common on the right side.

1.105

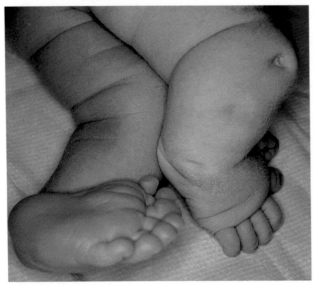

Figure 1.105. In the tibia reduction-polydactyly syndrome, the fibula may be shortened but is otherwise normal and the patella may be absent. Associated malformations are common and strikingly heterogeneous. Note the skin dimple at the knee joint and the skin dimple over the leg, and the bilateral pes equinovarus associated with the absence of the tibiae. The plantar surface of the foot is turned medially.

Skin dimples at a joint are seen normally in infants but dimples over a long bone are always associated with pathology.

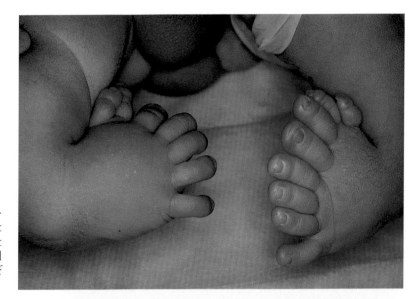

1.106

Figure 1.106. Tibia reduction-poly-dactyly syndrome in the same infant showing the septadactyly of the right foot, octadactyly of the left foot and bilateral pes equinovarus because of absence of the tibia.

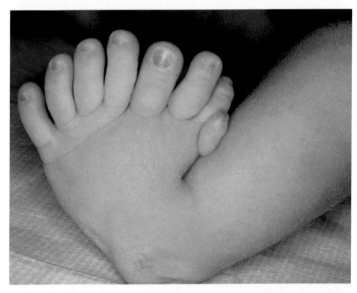

1.107

Figure 1.107. Octadactyly and pes equino-varus of the left foot in the same infant. Note the position of the big toe. The extra digits are therefore preaxial.

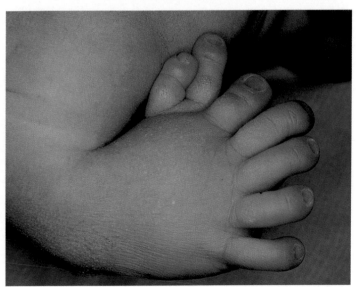

1.108

Figure 1.108. The same infant showing the septadactyly and pes equinovarus of the right foot. Note the position of the big toe. The extra digits are also preaxial.

1.109

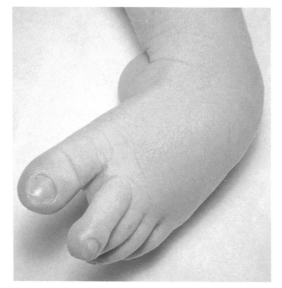

Figure 1.109. Talipes equinovarus (congenital clubfoot). There has been much discussion as to whether this is a true congenital malformation or whether it occurs as a result of a postural deformity (intrauterine molding). The foot cannot be dorsiflexed to the normal position and the heel is fixed in the varus deformity.

1.110

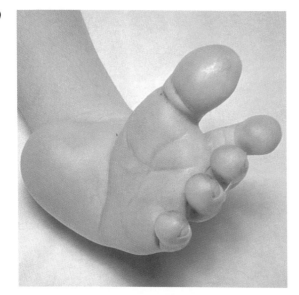

Figure 1.110. Another view of the foot of the same infant.

1.111

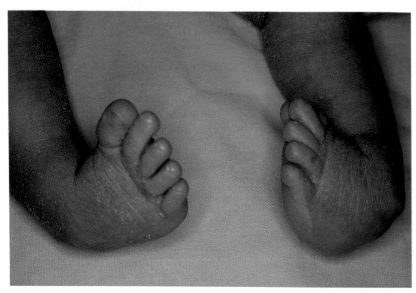

Figure 1.111. Talipes equinovarus (congenital clubfoot) in an infant with Poland's anomaly. Talipes equinovarus is frequently associated with congenital hip dysplasia, neural tube defects, and neuromuscular conditions.

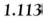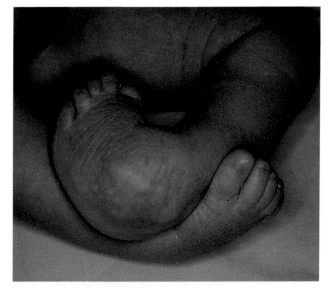

1.112

Figure 1.112. The same infant showing the position of the feet in utero, suggesting that the defect occurred as a result of a congenital postural deformity. In infants with clubfoot occurring as a congenital malformation, skin dimples are not present at the ankles, whereas in infants with clubfoot associated with postural deformations, dimples may be present over the joint as is noted in this infant.

1.113

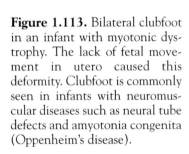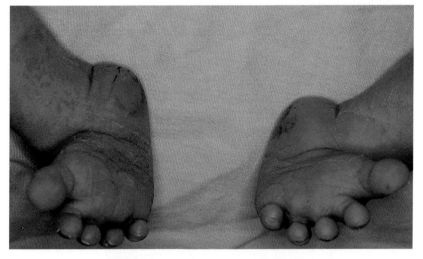

Figure 1.113. Bilateral clubfoot in an infant with myotonic dystrophy. The lack of fetal movement in utero caused this deformity. Clubfoot is commonly seen in infants with neuromuscular diseases such as neural tube defects and amyotonia congenita (Oppenheim's disease).

1.114

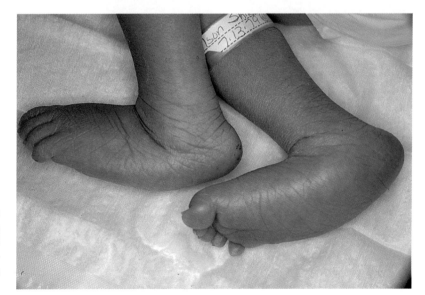

Figure 1.114. Rocker-bottom feet are noted in this infant with trisomy 18. Posterior calcaneal extension is present and the convex appearance of the sole of the foot resembles a "rocking chair."

1.115

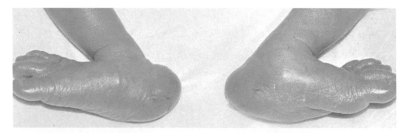

Figure 1.115. This infant with a neural tube defect presents a classic appearance of rocker-bottom feet with marked posterior calcaneal extension. Rocker-bottom feet are commonly seen in infants with neural tube defects.

1.116

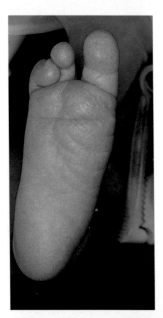
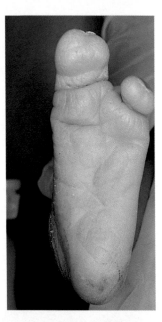

Figure 1.116. An example of ectrodactyly of both feet. Note that there are three toes on the right foot and three toes on the left foot with fusion of the first and second toes. The sole creases are poorly developed.

1.117

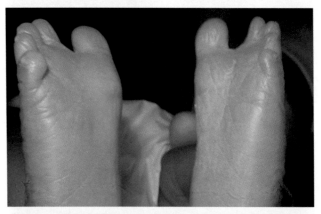

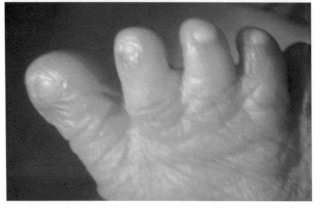

Figure 1.117. Microsyndactyly of the toes in an otherwise normal infant.

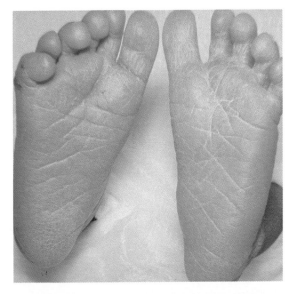

1.118

Figure 1.118. Polydactyly of toes of the right foot.

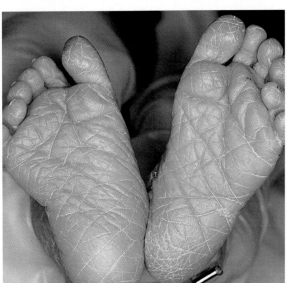

1.119

Figure 1.119. Polydactyly of the toes of both feet.

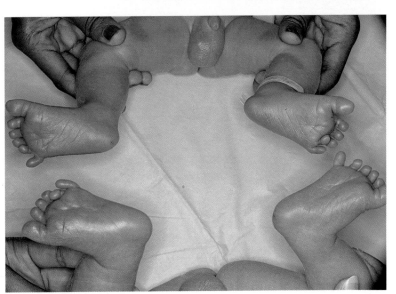

1.120

Figure 1.120. Bilateral polydactyly of toes in identical twins.

1.121

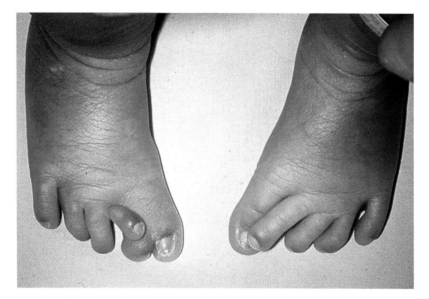

Figure 1.121. Central polydactyly and syndactyly of the first and second toes of the right foot in an infant of a diabetic mother. Otherwise, the infant was normal.

1.122

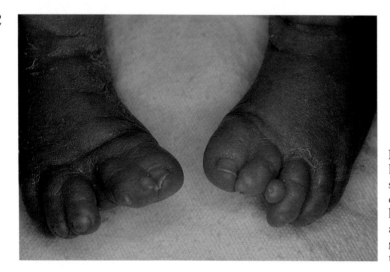

Figure 1.122. Central polydactyly of the left foot with syndactyly of the first and second toes of both feet. This infant, who clinically was not typical of a trisomy 18, had the radiographic findings of a gracile appearance of the ribs and an antimongoloid pelvis. The karyotype was a typical trisomy 18.

1.123

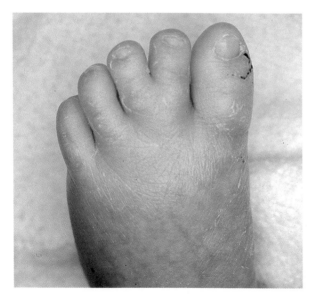

Figure 1.123. Syndactyly in an otherwise normal infant is of no medical or cosmetic significance and involves the toes more frequently than the fingers. Syndactyly refers to fusion of the soft tissues without synostosis. It is also seen in many syndromes such as Smith-Lemli-Opitz, Apert's, and trisomy 18.

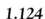

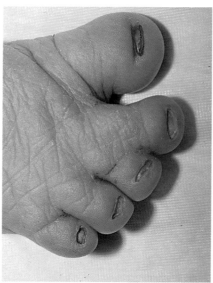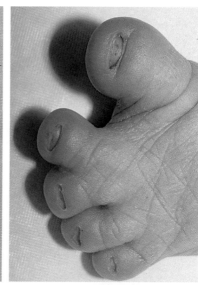

Figure 1.124. Syndactyly of the second and third toes bilaterally with markedly hypoplastic nails in an infant who also had a floating thumb of the right hand. Chromosomes were normal.

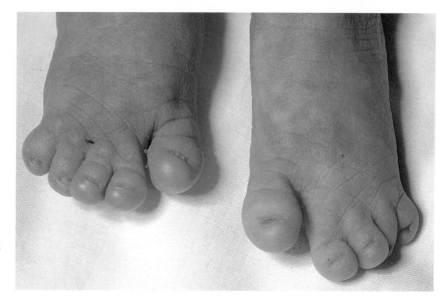

Figure 1.125. Mild syndactyly of the second and third toes in an infant with the other typical findings of trisomy 18, namely the short big toes and hypoplastic nails.

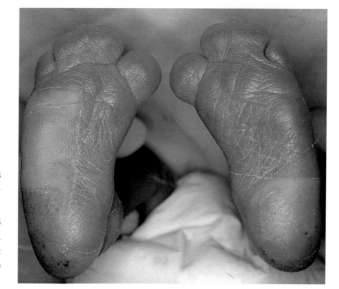

Figure 1.126. Symmetrical syndactyly of the toes in an infant with Apert's syndrome (acrocephalosyndactyly).

In symphalangism, no joint movement whatever is possible at the sites of the affected interphalangeal joints because the bony fusion has taken place. The absence of flexion creases is an excellent clue to the presence of this anomaly.

1.127

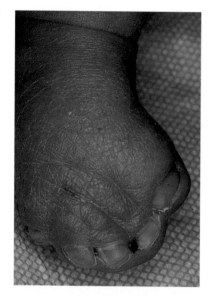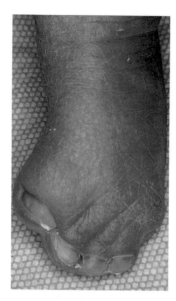

Figure 1.127. Another example of symmetrical syndactyly of the toes in Apert's syndrome.

1.128

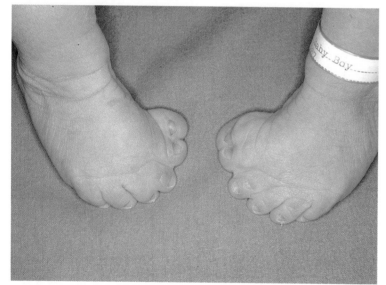

Figure 1.128. Bilateral symmetrical polysyndactyly giving the appearance of webbing between the toes in an infantwith Carpenter's syndrome (acrocephalopolysyndactyly).

1.129

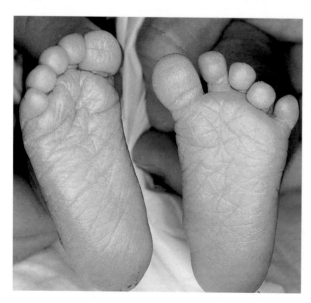

Figure 1.129. Broad toes in a normal infant. This may be familial. Broad toes are seen in certain syndromes such as Rubenstein-Taybi syndrome and Larsen's syndrome.

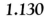

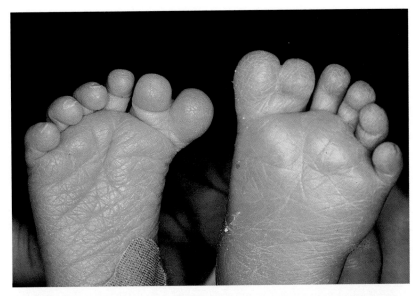

Figure 1.130. Preaxial polydactyly with bifid big toes in an otherwise normal infant.

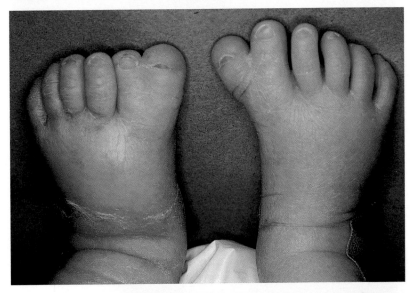

Figure 1.131. Bifid big toes with polydactyly in an infant who also has digitalization of the thumbs.

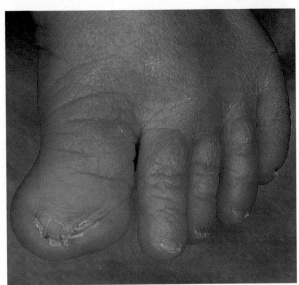

Figure 1.132. Duplication of the big toe. Radiograph showed two separate digits. This may result from an early insult to the limb bud in the 5th to 6th week of gestation.

1.133

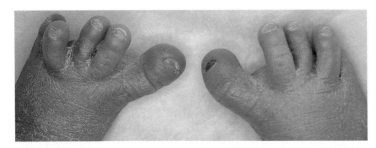

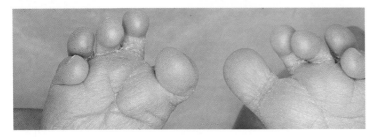

Figure 1.133. Congenital curly toes ("overlapping" toes). These are very common and are often familial. The abnormality becomes less obvious as the infant grows.

1.134

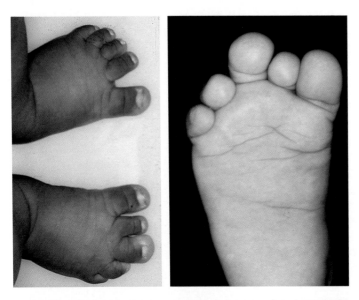

Figure 1.134. Hypertrophy of the third toe of the right foot. This may occur as an isolated finding or may be seen in neurofibromatosis or in infants with vascular malformation of a digit.

1.135

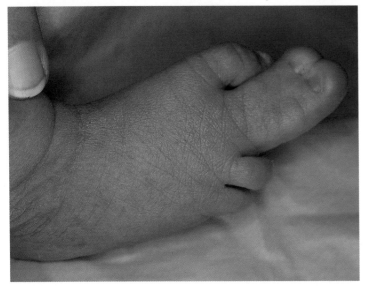

Figure 1.135. Dorsal view of macrosyndactyly of the second and third toes of the right foot.

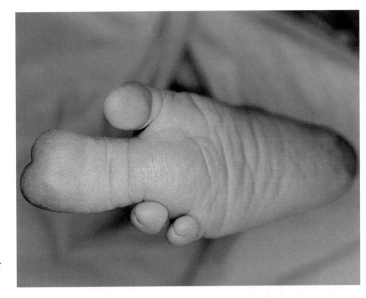

Figure 1.136. Plantar view of the toes of the same infant.

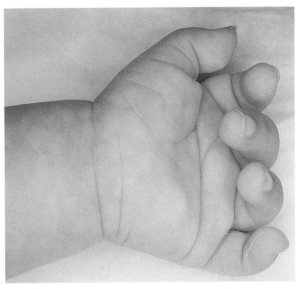

Figure 1.137. Single palmar crease and clinodactyly in the left hand of an otherwise normal infant. Single palmar creases are noted bilaterally in 1 to 2% of normal infants and unilaterally in 6% of normal infants. It is present in about 50% of patients with Down syndrome. It is twice as common in males as in females and it is associated with many syndromes. Palm creases form in response to flexion at the metacarpophalangeal joints and opposition of the thumb. Three deep creases are usually seen but there are many normal variants.

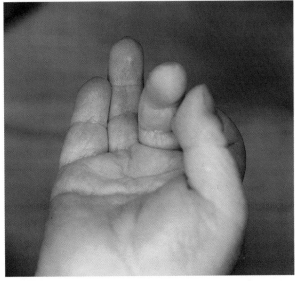

Figure 1.138. Single palmar crease and clinodactyly of the right hand. Clinodactyly is the incurving of the finger to one side, usually toward the midline, due to an absent or hypoplastic middle phalanx. Involvement of the fifth finger is most common. With an absent phalanx only two creases are present as in this infant. With a hypoplastic middle phalanx, the number of creases is normal but creases are closer together and will slope toward each other rather than being parallel. It is noted in otherwise normal infants but also occurs in many syndromes.

1.139

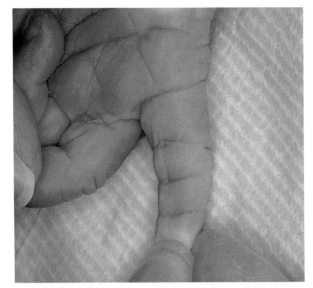

Figure 1.139. An extra crease on the fifth finger.

1.140

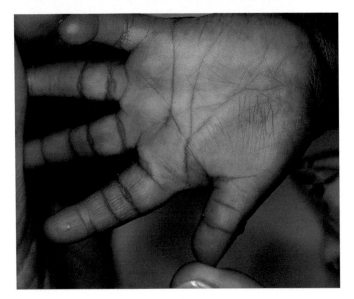

Figure 1.140. Increased number of finger creases in an otherwise normal infant. Increased finger creases may be seen in normal infants and in infants that have increased laxity of the joints such as in Larsen's syndrome and Ehlers-Danlos syndrome. They often signify increased fetal activity at 11 to 12 weeks of fetal life when the creases normally become evident. Hence, gross alteration in crease patterning is usually indicative of an abnormality in form and/or function of the hand prior to the 11th fetal week. If there is a lack of fetal movement before this period of gestation, the number of finger creases is decreased.

1.141

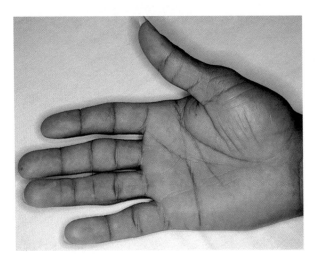

Figure 1.141. The father of the same infant also had increased finger creases. He was otherwise normal and had no problems. The thenar crease normally circles the base of the thenar eminence, extending distally to between the thumb and index fingers. The distal palmar crease traverses the palm beneath the last three fingers, beginning at the ulnar edge of the palm and curving distally to exit between the middle and index fingers. The proximal palmar crease may be less well defined. It begins over the hypothenar eminence and normally extends parallel to the distal crease to exit near or fuse with the distal portion of the thenar crease.

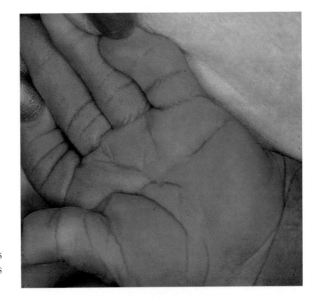

1.142

Figure 1.142. Increased and abnormal finger creases due to laxity of joints in an infant with Larsen's syndrome. Note the single palmar crease.

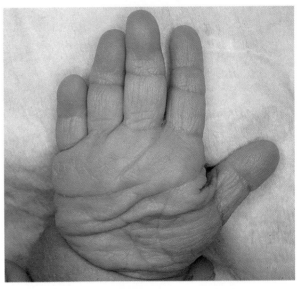

1.143

Figure 1.143. This infant has decreased creases in both the fingers and the palm due to lack of fetal movement. Absence of normal flexion creases invariably signifies inadequate movement of the underlying joints. Changes in the palmar crease include the single palmar crease (simian crease) and the bridged palmar crease (Sydney line) in which there is an extension of the proximal transverse crease which reaches the ulnar border of the hand and the medial edge of the palm between the index and middle fingers.

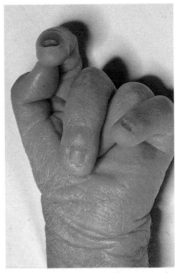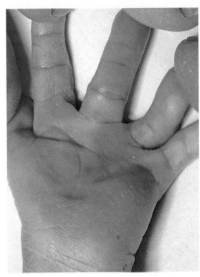

1.144

Figure 1.144. Lack of fetal movement is seen in acute infantile spinal atrophy (Werdnig-Hoffmann disease). Lack of normal development of the finger creases is due to lack of fetal movement early in gestation. On the left, note the position of comfort of the fingers with deep depression in the palm shown on the right.

1.145

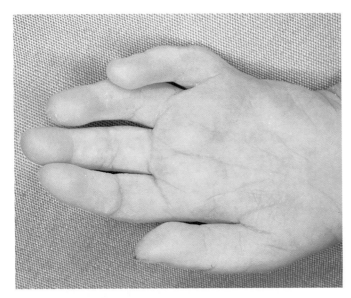

Figure 1.145. Lack of creases of the palm and fingers in an infant with amyotonia congenita.

1.146

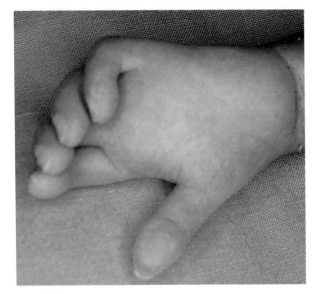

Figure 1.146. Hypoplastic (absent or sparse) dermal ridges and absence of flexion creases on the fingers and palms are seen in this infant with the fetal akinesia sequence (Pena-Shokeir phenotype).

1.147

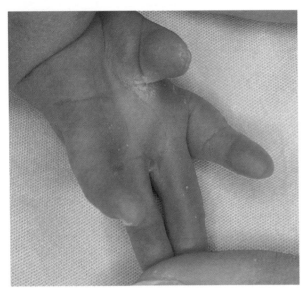

Figure 1.147. This infant with arthrogryposis multiplex congenita shows the lack of palmar and finger creases due to lack of fetal movement before the 10th to 12th weeks of gestation.

1.148

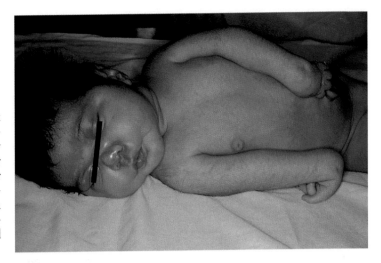

Figure 1.148. Arthrogryposis multiplex congenita in this infant shows the contractures which occur in this condition. They are usually symmetrical and involve all four extremities but may involve only the upper or lower limbs. There is muscular hypotonia, generalized thickening of the skin with dimpling, and hip subluxation; and bilateral talipes equinovarus, opisthotonos and scoliosis of the spine are common.

1.149

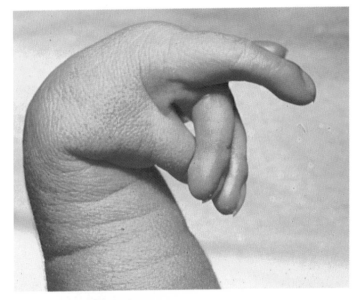

Figure 1.149. Contracture of the hand in an infant with arthrogryposis multiplex congenita.

1.150

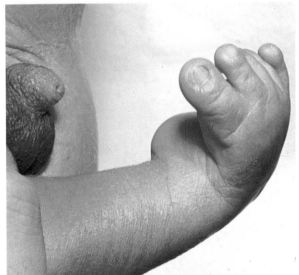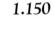

Figure 1.150. Contracture of the lower extremity in the same infant. These infants commonly have bilateral talipes equinovarus.

1.151

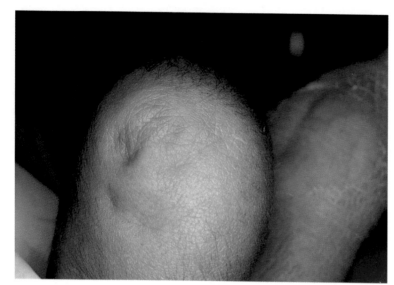

Figure 1.151. Dimples at the knee in an infant with arthrogryposis multiplex congenita. Normally dimples at a joint are of no significance, but they may occur with contractures and lack of movement as in this infant.

Chapter 2
Dwarfism

Dwarfs frequently present in the newborn period, but sometimes the diagnosis is not obvious until there is additional disproportionate growth. There are many different kinds of dwarfs and the nomenclature is descriptive of the portions of the long bones affected. Rhizomelic shortening refers to the proximal portions of the long bones (e.g., upper arms and thighs). Mesomelic shortening refers to the central segments of the long bones (e.g., forearms and legs). Acromelic shortening refers to the hands and feet. All three segments may be affected simultaneously but unequally, as in achondroplasia in which the most severe effect is in the proximal segment. All four limbs may be involved as in Conradi-Hünermann syndrome. Only the femur may be involved as in femoral hypoplasia syndrome or only the forearms may be affected as in Robinow's syndrome. A general knowledge of the various kinds of dwarfs is important in their recognition. Frequently, consultation with a radiologist, geneticist, pediatrician or neonatologist experienced in recognizing dwarfs may be necessary.

2.1

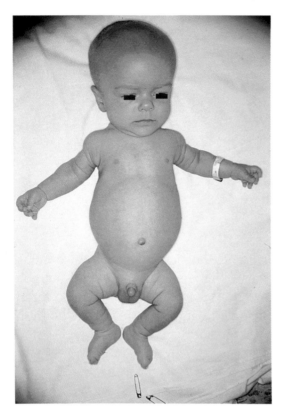

Figure 2.1. Achondroplasia (rhizomelic dwarfism). This is dominantly inherited but many cases occur by spontaneous mutation. There are short proximal parts of the arms and legs (rhizomelic micromelia), marked lordosis, caudal narrowing of the spine, and spade-like hands (short "trident" hand with short metacarpals and phalanges). Note the normally sized but laterally compressed trunk.

2.2

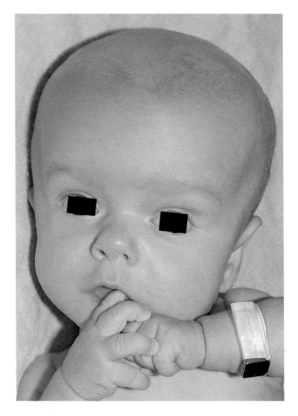

Figure 2.2. The head of the same infant showing the large square head with bossing of the forehead and a depressed nasal bridge. Infants with achondroplasia may have megalencephaly (macroencephaly).

In hypochondroplasia syndrome there is a near normal craniofacies but the limbs are short and there is caudal narrowing of the spine.

2.3

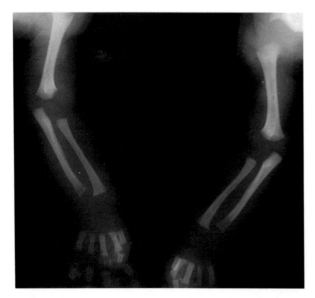

Figure 2.3. A radiograph of the upper extremities showing the short proximal parts. Note that the typical changes in the long bones are not yet present.

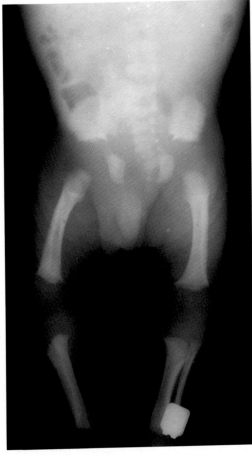

2.4

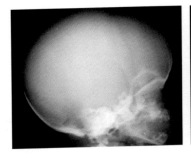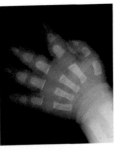

2.5

Figure 2.5. Radiograph of skull on the left showing the large size, shortened base and shallow sella turcica. This is characteristic in achondroplasia. On the right is a radiograph of the left hand showing the broad and short bones.

Figure 2.4. A radiograph of the lower extremities showing the short proximal parts. Note that the bones are broad and short.

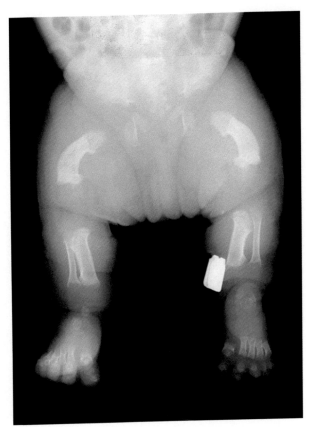

2.6

Figure 2.6. A radiograph of the lower extremities in an infant with achondroplasia. Note the broad short bones with irregular and flared epiphyseal lines. Note the typical "telephone handle" appearance of the femur.

2.7

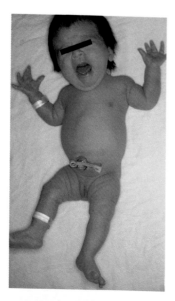

Figure 2.7. Another example of achondroplasia in a term infant. The infant's length was 45 cm with an upper/lower segment ratio of 2.3. The upper/lower segment ratio for a term infant is 1.7. The shortness of length and the increase in upper/lower segment ratio is due to the short lower extremities. The head circumference of 36 cm is above the 90th percentile.

2.8

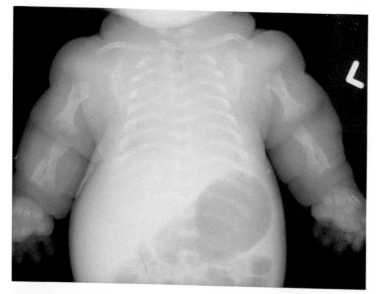

Figure 2.8. A radiograph of an infant with achondroplasia. Note the rhizomelic upper extremities and the narrow ribs which result in compression of the chest.

2.9

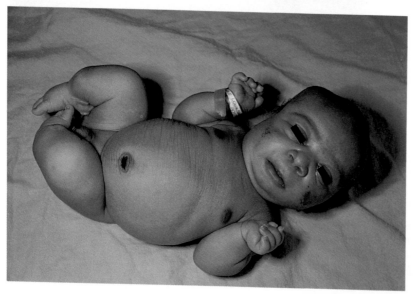

Figure 2.9. Camptomelic dysplasia. Note the short limbs and marked bowing of the tibiae in this autosomal recessive type of dwarfism. The infants have a flat facies with a low nasal bridge and micrognathia. The majority of infants die in the neonatal period from respiratory insufficiency.

2.10

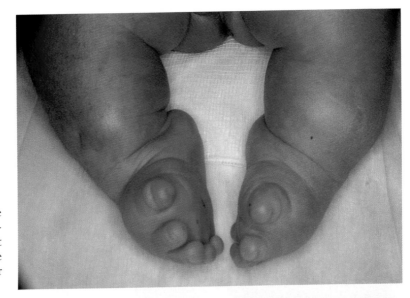

Figure 2.10. Note the bowed tibiae and the skin dimple over the midportion of the leg in the same infant with camptomelic dysplasia. These occur as a result of absent or hypoplastic fibulae in these infants.

2.11

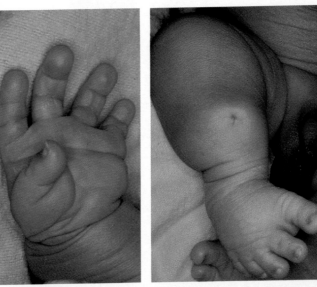

Figure 2.11. The same infant showing the left hand and the right leg. Note the short stubby fingers,   single palmar crease and clinodactyly of the fifth finger and the anterior bowing of the tibia with skin dimpling over the convex area. Dimples at a joint are common and usually normal but the presence of skin dimples between joints, such as in this infant, always signifies underlying pathology.

2.12

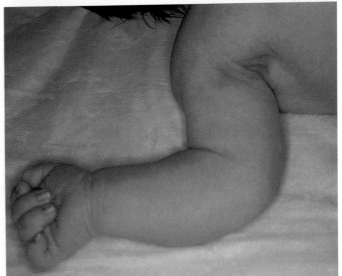

Figure 2.12. Note the marked shortening of the proximal portion of the right upper extremity compared with the distal portion in an infant with camptomelic dysplasia.

2.13

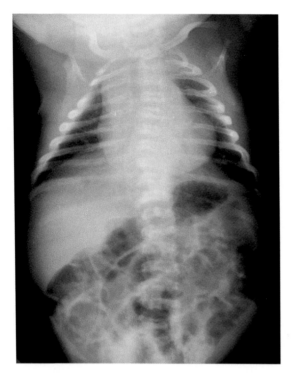

Figure 2.13. A radiograph of the chest of this infant shows the small thoracic cage with thin, short clavicles and hypoplastic scapulae. This is a typical finding in camptomelic dysplasia.

2.14

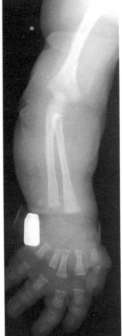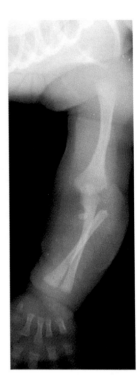

Figure 2.14. Radiograph of the upper extremities of the same infant with camptomelic dysplasia showing the hypoplastic scapulae, bowing of long bones, radioulnar dislocation and short proximal phalanges.

2.15

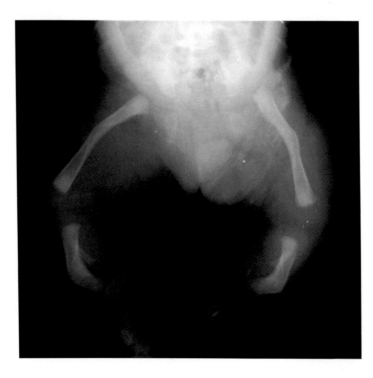

Figure 2.15. Radiograph of the lower extremities of the same infant with camptomelic dysplasia. Note the marked bowing of the long bones with cortical thickening of the concave border and thinning of the convex border. Also note the absent left fibula and hypoplastic right fibula.

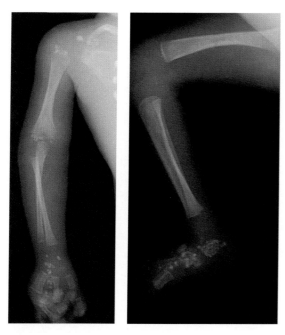 2.16

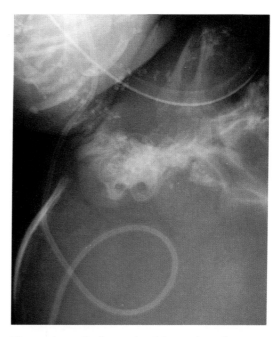 2.17

Figure 2.16. Radiograph of the upper and lower extremities showing the stippling of the epiphyses of an infant with chondrodystrophia calcificans congenita. This may occur as a rhizomelic form with a flat facies, low nasal bridge and cataracts, short humeri and femora, coronal clefts in the vertebrae, and punctate epiphyseal mineralization. It also occurs in an autosomal dominant form (Conradi-Hünermann syndrome) in which there is asymmetric limb shortness and early punctate epiphyseal mineralization. In infants with stippling of the epiphyses, consideration should also be given to the diagnoses of Zellweger syndrome and the fetal warfarin syndrome.

Figure 2.17. Radiograph of the neck in the same infant showing the characteristic stippling at the hyoid bone and the spine.

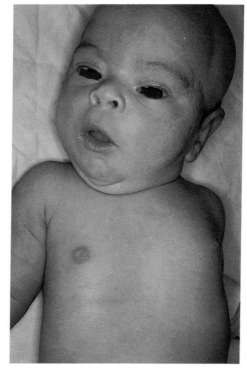 2.18

Figure 2.18. In this infant with cleidocranial dysplasia, an autosomal dominant condition, the shoulders clinically appear normal. They may present with hanging narrow shoulders, pectus excavatum, and abnormal shoulder movement due to the bilateral absence of the clavicles. In any infant with wide open sutures and fontanelles or wormian bones on clinical examination of the skull, one should always check the clavicles to exclude the diagnosis of cleidocranial dysostosis.

2.19

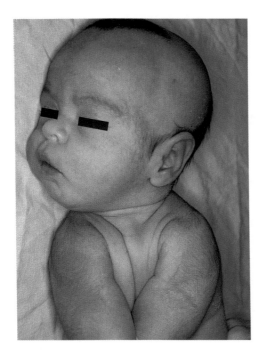

Figure 2.19. The same infant as in Figure 2.18 with cleidocranial dysplasia showing the approximation of the shoulders in front of the chest due to the absence of the clavicles. These infants present with other findings. Aplasia or defective development of the clavicles and laxity of the ligaments allow the forward folding of the shoulders. Defective mineralization of other parts of the skeleton may occur.

2.20

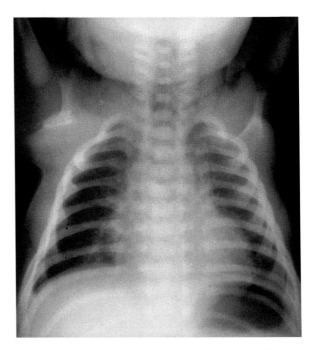

Figure 2.20. Radiograph of the chest shows the absence of the clavicles.

2.21

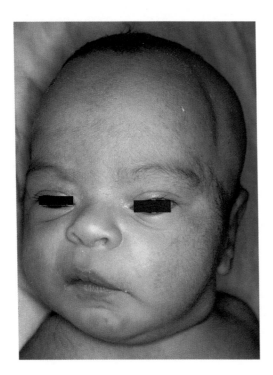

Figure 2.21. This figure shows the same infant with frontal and parietal bossing. The face appears small with a broad nose and depressed nasal bridge, and there is a groove over the metopic suture. The infant also had a large, open fontanelle.

2.22

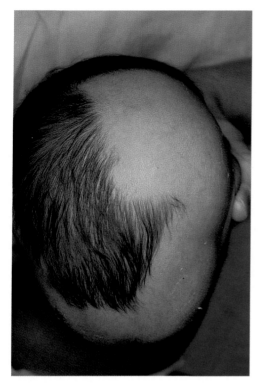

Figure 2.22. The same infant showing the brachycephalic skull and frontal and parietal bossing.

2.23

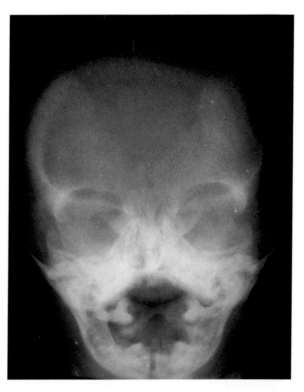

Figure 2.23. The radiograph of the skull in the same infant. Note the wide open fontanelles due to their delayed closure. There is also marked widening of the cranial sutures.

2.24

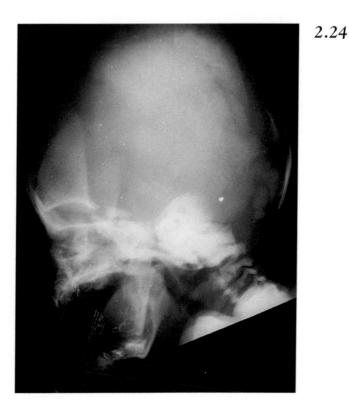

Figure 2.24. A lateral radiograph of the skull in an infant with cleidocranial dysostosis showing the marked frontal and parietal bossing and brachycephaly.

2.25

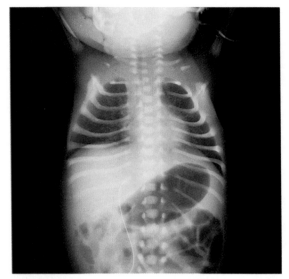

Figure 2.25. This infant with cleidocranial dysostosis has hypoplastic clavicles and had the typical findings in the skull. In cleidocranial dysostosis there may be partial to complete dysplasia of the clavicles.

2.26

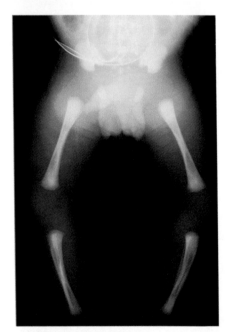

Figure 2.26. The radiograph of the pelvis and long bones of the same infant shows the poorly developed pelvis with small ilia and marked separation of the symphysis pubis.

2.27

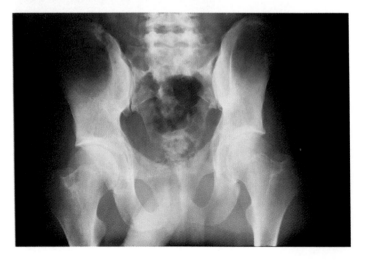

Figure 2.27. Radiograph of the pelvis of the father of the same infant at the age of 25 years. Note the retarded ossification of the corpora and inferior rami of the pubic bones and the retarded ossification of the symphysis pubis (i.e., symphysis pubis gap is not fused).

2.28

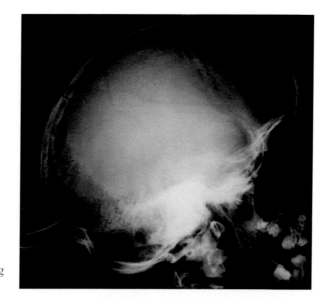

Figure 2.28. Radiograph of the father's skull showing the poor ossification and multiple wormian bones.

2.29

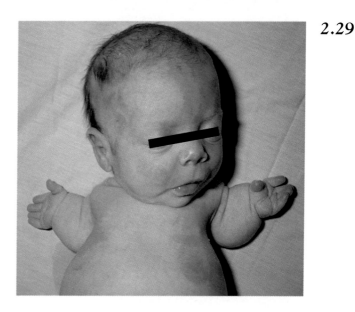

Figure 2.29. This infant with diastrophic dysplasia presents the marked narrowing of the chest, the short limbs and the typical "hitchhiker" thumbs (hyperextensible and hyperabductable). In this autosomal recessive condition there is disproportionate dwarfism (abnormal shortness of the proximal parts of the limbs), club feet, and widening between the first and second toes ("sandal" sign). The big toes are abducted.

2.30

Figure 2.30. This figure is a close-up of the typical "hitchhiker" thumbs in the same infant with diastrophic dysplasia. The "hitchhiker" thumb is caused by hypoplasia of the first metacarpal, and the long axis of the digit is oriented almost horizontally in relation to the palm. The thumb is retroflexed with hypoplasia of the thenar musculature. Radiographic examination of the long bones in these infants demonstrates spreading of the metaphyses and delayed closure and deformation of the epiphyses.

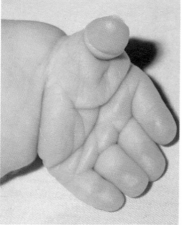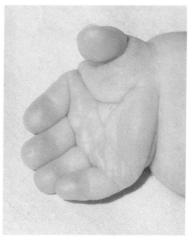

2.31

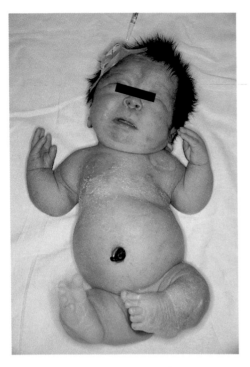

2.32

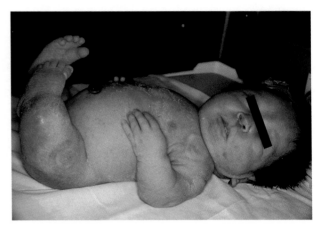

Figure 2.32. A lateral view of the same infant.

Figure 2.31. This infant has a rare form of short-limbed dwarfism. The diagnosis is anisospondylic camptomicromelic dwarfism (dyssegmental dwarfism). This condition is autosomal recessive, there is disproportionate short stature, flat facies, flat nose and micrognathia. Cleft palate is common. There is a short neck and narrow thorax with short bent extremities and decreased joint mobility. A radiograph of the spine is diagnostic in that there are short vertebral bodies with segmentation defects.

2.33

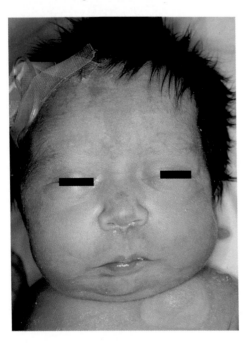

Figure 2.33. A close-up view of the same infant showing the flat facies with a flat nose, micrognathia and a short neck.

2.34

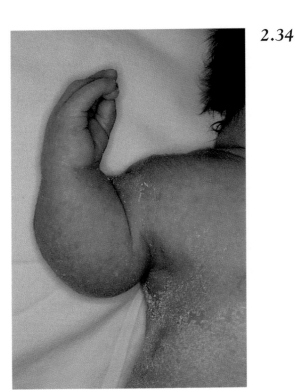

2.35

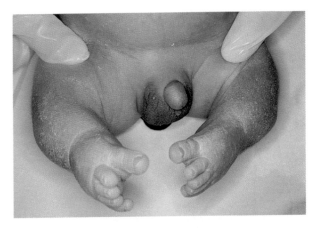

Figure 2.35. The lower extremities of the same infant showing the marked camptomicromelia.

Figure 2.34. The right upper extremity of the same infant showing the camptomicromelia and the small thorax.

2.36

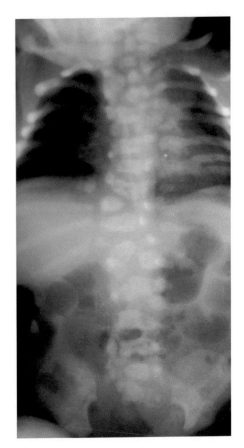

Figure 2.36. Radiograph of the chest and spine of the same infant with dyssegmental dwarfism. Note the anisospondyly (segmentation defects of the vertebral bodies), abnormalities of the ribs, hypoplastic scapulae, and ilia with irregular borders.

2.37

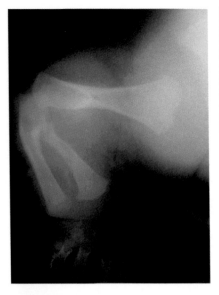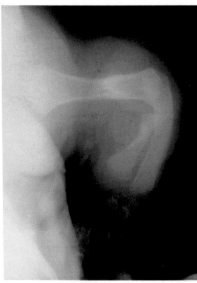

Figure 2.37. Radiograph of the upper extremities of the same infant as in Figure 2.31 showing the long bones which are markedly shortened with midshaft angulation (camptomelia) together with marked metaphyseal flaring and cupping.

2.38

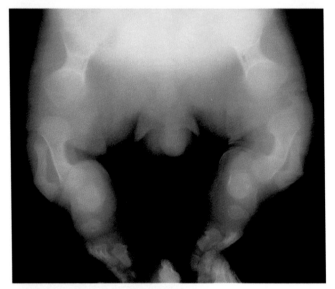

Figure 2.38. Radiograph of the lower extremities of the same infant. The long bones are markedly shortened with midshaft angulation (camptomelia) together with marked metaphyseal flaring and cupping.

2.39

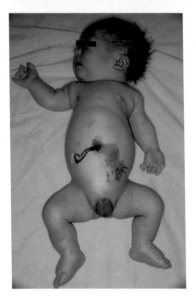

Figure 2.39. This infant with chondroectodermal dysplasia (Ellis-van Creveld syndrome) presents with the typical short distal extremities, short ribs, polydactyly, nail hypoplasia, neonatal teeth, and congenital heart disease. Although atrial septal defect is most common, this infant had a hypoplastic left heart. Note that the extremities are plump and markedly and progressively shortened distally, that is, from the trunk to the phalanges. Birthweight was 2880 g, length was 44.5 cm (<10th percentile), and fronto-occipital circumference (FOC) was 34.5 cm (50th percentile).

2.40

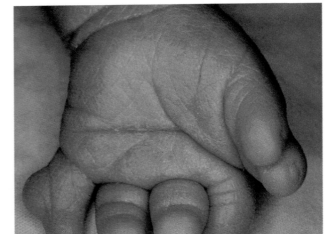

Figure 2.40. A close-up of the left hand of the infant shown in Figure 2.39 showing polydactyly (seven digits) and brachydactyly.

2.41

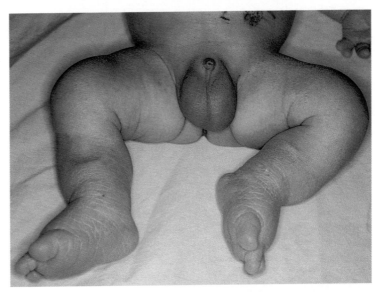

Figure 2.41. Note the typical lower extremities in the same infant. The limbs which are short and plump become markedly and progressively shortened distally, that is, from the trunk to the phalanges. Also note the very small penis (genital anomalies are not uncommon in this condition).

2.42

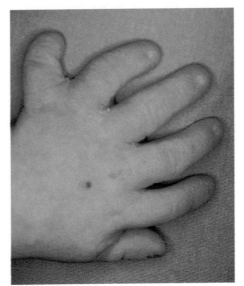

Figure 2.42. Preaxial polydactyly and brachydactyly in another infant with Ellis-van Creveld syndrome. Note the markedly hypoplastic nails.

2.43

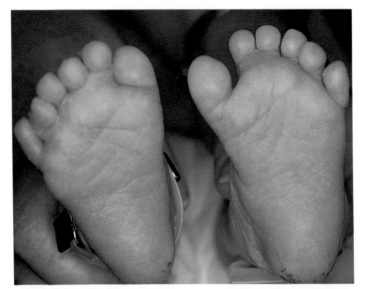

Figure 2.43. Postaxial polydactyly of the toes in an infant with Ellis-van Creveld syndrome. In this syndrome, polydactyly is noted in the fingers in 100% of cases but is present in the toes in only 10 to 20%.

2.44

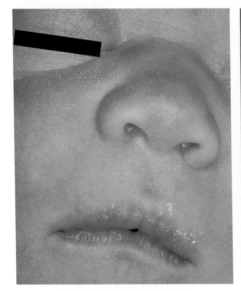

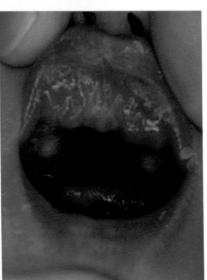

Figure 2.44. In this infant with Ellis-van Creveld syndrome, note on the left the short upper lip with midline defect due to fusion of the upper lip to the maxillary-gingival margin. On the right, note that the fusion of the upper lip to the maxillary-gingival margin results in a lack of the mucobuccal fold or sulcus which normally is present anteriorly.

2.45

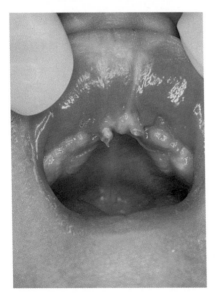

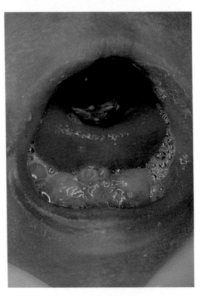

Figure 2.45. This infant with Ellis-van Creveld syndrome demonstrates on the left the fusion of the labiogingival margins so there is no sulcus to the upper lip. Also note the hypoplastic neonatal teeth in the upper jaw. On the right, note the hypoplastic neonatal teeth in the lower jaw. Neonatal teeth are present in 30% of infants with Ellis-van Creveld syndrome.

2.46

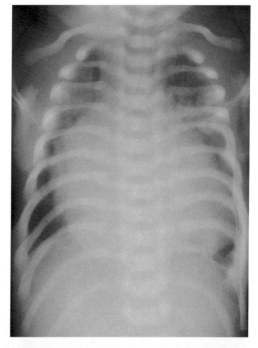

Figure 2.46. A radiograph of the chest of an infant with Ellis-van Creveld syndrome. Note the long narrow chest and short ribs with cardiac enlargement. Congenital heart disease is present in 50 to 60% of cases of Ellis-van Creveld syndrome. This infant had a large atrial septal defect, the most common lesion seen in Ellis-van Creveld syndrome.

2.47

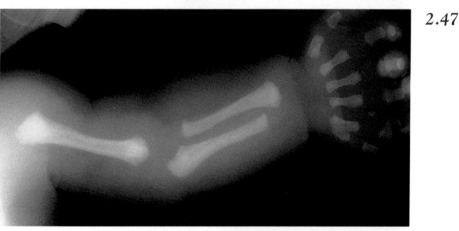

Figure 2.47. Radiograph showing the mesomelic shortening of the limbs and polydactyly. The proximal end of the ulna and distal end of the radius are swollen and bulbous giving the appearance of two parallel drumsticks that point in opposite directions.

2.48

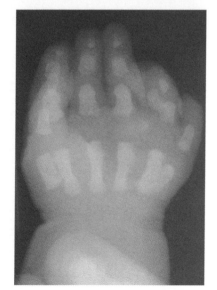

Figure 2.48. Radiograph of the hand in an infant with Ellis-van Creveld syndrome. Note that the phalanges are short but that the proximal phalanges are relatively long compared to the others. Adults, therefore, cannot make a tight fist. Also note the fusion of the fifth and sixth metacarpals.

2.49

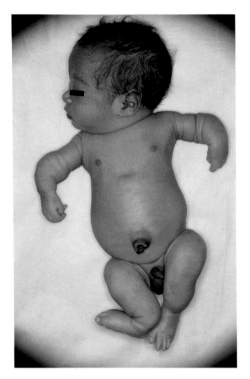

2.50

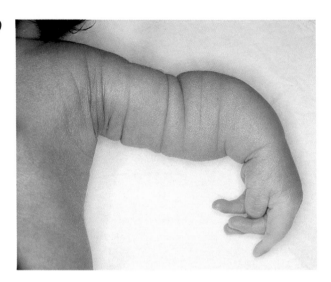

Figure 2.50. Close-up view of the arm of the same infant showing the marked bowing at the forearm.

Figure 2.49. Short-limbed dwarfism in an infant with congenital hypophosphatasia. There is failure of calcification of all bones resulting in marked bowing. This autosomal recessive condition is associated with a severe deficiency of tissue and serum alkaline phosphatase. It presents with bowed lower extremities with overlying cutaneous dimpling and short ribs resulting in a small thoracic cage. Death usually occurs from respiratory insufficiency.

2.51

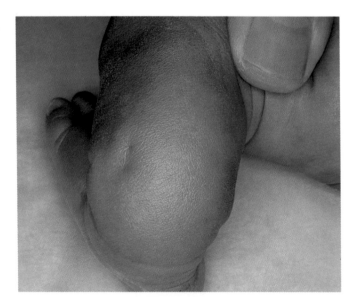

Figure 2.51. The lower right leg of the same infant showing the marked bowing with a large skin dimple over the middle of the leg. This is a classic physical sign in infants with congenital hypophosphatasia.

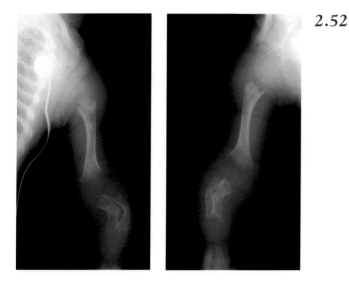

Figure 2.52. Radiograph of the upper extremity showing the osteoporosis and metaphyseal flaring with marked bowing of the radius and ulna bilaterally.

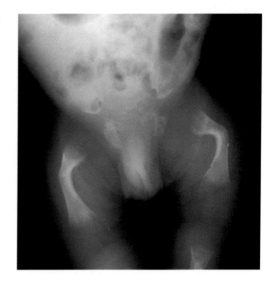

Figure 2.53. Radiograph of the lower extremities of the same infant showing the gross osteoporosis and metaphyseal flaring with marked bowing of the femora, tibiae and fibulae.

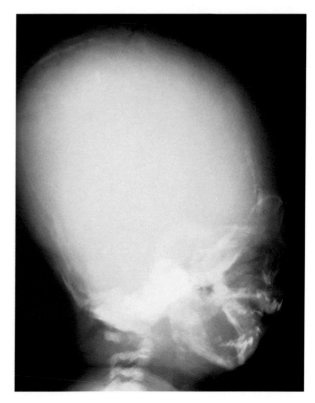

Figure 2.54. Radiograph of the skull of an infant with congenital hypophosphatasia. Note the marked lack of mineralization with deformity of the skull. Characteristic is the large size of the skull, shortened base, and a shallow sella turcica. There is late closure of the fontanelles. This appearance is comparable to the skull seen in infants with osteogenesis imperfecta.

2.55

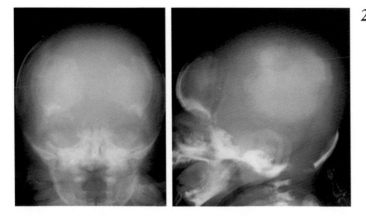

Figure 2.55. Radiograph of the skull of another infant with congenital hypophosphatasia. Note that some mineralization is present but that it is very poor.

2.56

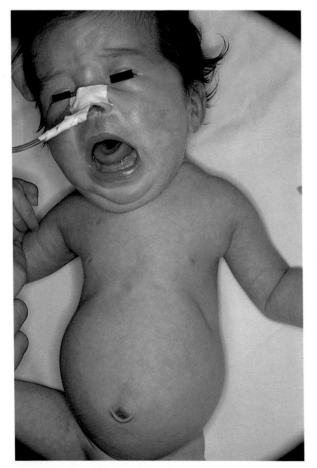

Figure 2.56. In this infant with asphyxiating thoracic dystrophy (Jeune's syndrome) note the abnormally long and narrow thorax with high clavicles and a large abdomen. The narrow thorax due to short ribs results in limited chest wall movement. As a result of this, there is a lack of space in the subcostal area and the liver lies completely in the abdomen. These infants may have hypoplastic lungs and renal pathology in the form of cystic tubular hypoplasia and/or glomerular sclerosis.

2.57

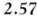

Figure 2.57. Another infant with asphyxiating thoracic dystrophy. Again note the small thorax due to short ribs, the high clavicles and what appears to be abdominal distention due to the fact that the whole liver is in the abdomen. These infants give the appearance of having widely spaced nipples. There is shortening of the arms and legs as well as an inability to extend the forearm at the elbow joint. The condition is autosomal recessive.

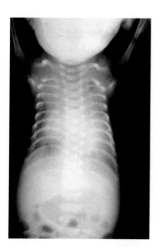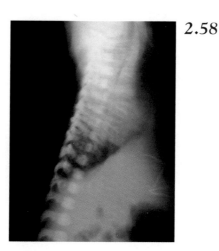

2.58

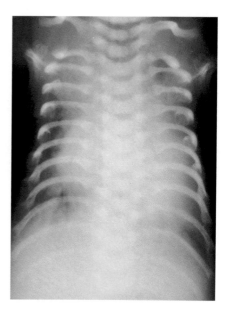

2.59

Figure 2.58. Anteroposterior and lateral radiograph of an infant with asphyxiating thoracic dystrophy. Note the short ribs which are horizontally placed, giving the appearance of a long narrow chest. The heart is normal in size but appears to be large because of the narrow thorax. Note the high clavicles, which are of normal size.

Figure 2.59. Radiograph of an infant with asphyxiating thoracic dystrophy. Note the very short ribs with a long narrow chest and the high clavicles.

2.60

Figure 2.60. Radiograph of the pelvis of an infant with asphyxiating thoracic dystrophy. Note the hypoplastic iliac wings and flattened acetabula with spike-like projections at the lower margins of the sciatic notches.

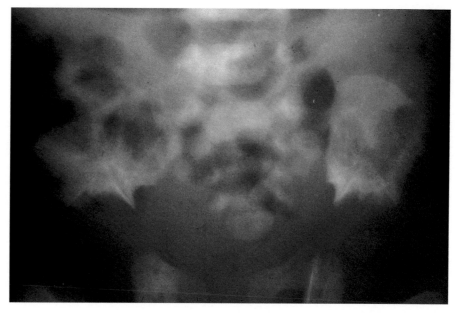

2.61

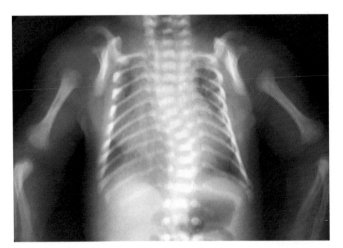

Figure 2.61. Radiograph of an infant with metatropic dysplasia. This is another form of dwarfism associated with a narrow thorax, thoracic kyphoscoliosis and metaphyseal flaring (giving the typical "dumb-bell" appearance). The proportion of the length of the trunk to the extremities reverses during childhood. At first the trunk is too long and the extremities too short. With increasing kyphoscoliosis the trunk becomes short.

2.62

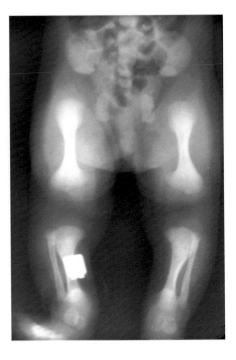

Figure 2.62. Radiograph of the lower extremities of the same infant showing the short limbs with typical "dumb-bell" appearance of the femora, which occurs as a result of huge epiphyses. There is hypoplasia of the basilar pelvis with horizontal acetabula, a short, deep sacroiliac notch, and squared iliac wings.

2.63

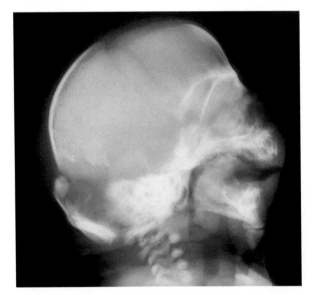

Figure 2.63. Radiograph of skull in an infant with metatropic dysplasia. Note the poor mineralization and the very prominent occiput.

2.64

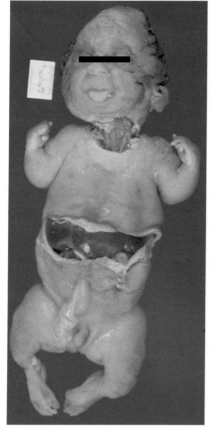

Figure 2.64. Type II osteogenesis imperfecta which is perinatally lethal. Death occurs before or shortly after birth. The lethal form is autosomally dominant but they are mostly new mutations. Rarely it is autosomally recessive. Note the markedly abnormal skull (which is soft and impressionable) and short limbs due to osteogenesis imperfecta. The damage to the neck and abdomen was present at birth.

2.65

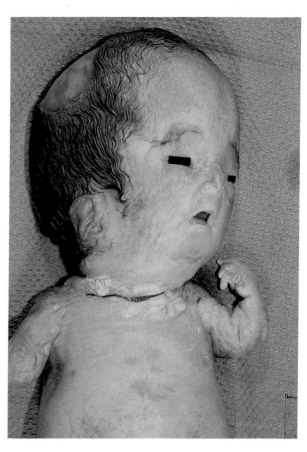

Figure 2.65. Another infant with severe osteogenesis imperfecta with marked shortening of long bones due to multiple fractures in utero as seen in the upper extremities and a grossly abnormal hand. This infant is another example of type II osteogenesis imperfecta. The head is grossly abnormal. The ear is not truly low set but gives this appearance due to the abnormal skull.

2.66

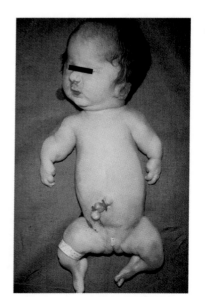

Figure 2.66. This infant with short extremities due to multiple in utero fractures is an example of type III osteogenesis imperfecta. The head is slightly enlarged, giving the ears a low-set appearance.

2.67

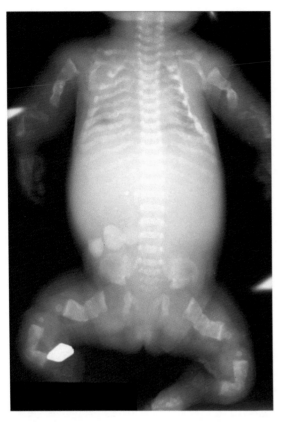

Figure 2.67. Total body radiograph of the same infant as in Figure 2.66 showing the numerous intrauterine fractures of the long bones of the extremities resulting in shortening of the extremities, and the intrauterine fractures of the ribs resulting in a narrow chest. Note the density above the right side of the pelvis. This is the umbilical cord stump which appears as an opacity in an abdominal radiograph where gas is lacking in the gastrointestinal tract.

2.68

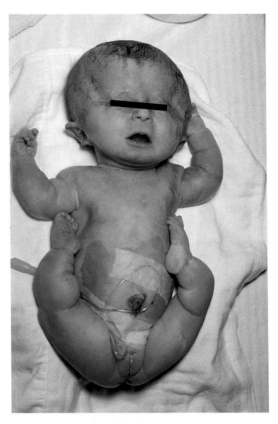

Figure 2.68. Another example of type III osteogenesis imperfecta showing the bowing and shortening of limbs due to intrauterine fractures. The skull is large and abnormal due to the lack of mineralization and multiple wormian bones. This infant also has a narrow chest due to intrauterine fractures of the ribs.

2.69

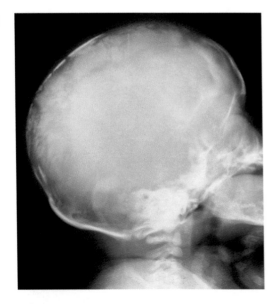

Figure 2.69. Radiograph of the skull in an infant with osteogenesis imperfecta. Note the lack of mineralization with wormian bones. Clinically one feels multiple small bones over the skull. There is a thin cortex with minimal skull ossification and generalized osteoporosis.

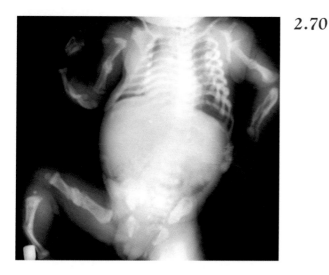

2.70

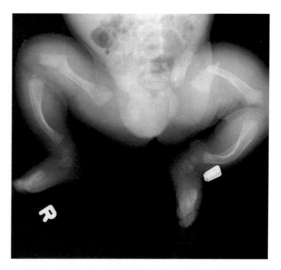

2.71

Figure 2.70. Another radiograph of an infant with type III osteogenesis imperfecta. Note the intrauterine fractures and bowing of the long bones.

Figure 2.71. Radiograph of osteogenesis imperfecta in a neonate. Note the fracture of the proximal part of the left femur and the marked bowing of the other long bones. This alerts one to the fact that mild forms of osteogenesis imperfecta may occur.

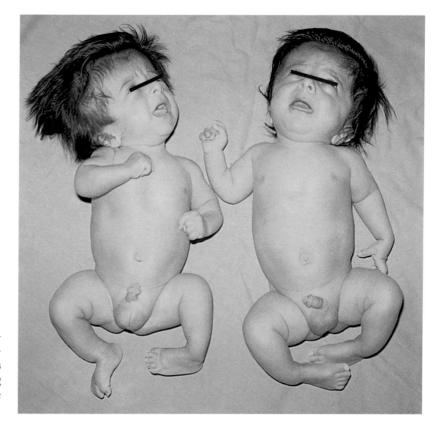

2.72

Figure 2.72. Type III osteogenesis imperfecta in identical twins. Note the large heads and the bowing of the long bones due to mild intrauterine fractures.

2.73

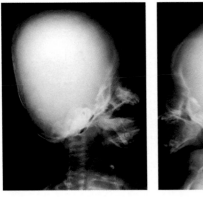

Figure 2.73. Radiograph of the skulls of the same twins as in Figure 2.72 showing the marked lack of mineralization.

2.74

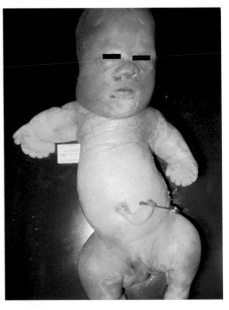

Figure 2.74. Short-limbed dwarfism in an infant with the Saldino-Noonan syndrome. This infant demonstrates the marked narrowing of the thorax with a large abdomen. The large abdomen is commonly seen in infants with a narrow thorax because the subcostal space is too small to accommodate the liver. The abdomen, per se, is normal. In this form of short-limbed dwarfism there is a narrow chest, due to short ribs, and polydactyly. (Richardson MM, Beaudet AL, Wanger ML, Malinis Rosenberg HS, Lucci JL: Prenatal diagnosis of recurrence of Saldino-Noonan dwarfism. *J. Pediatr* 91: 467-471. Reprinted with permission from Mosby Year Book, Inc., St. Louis, MO.)

2.75

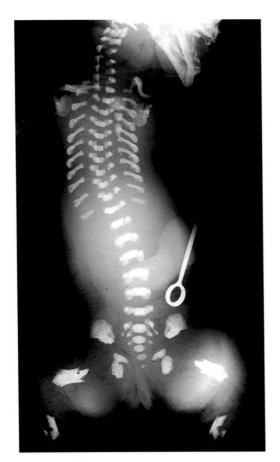

Figure 2.75. Body radiograph of an infant with Saldino-Noonan syndrome. In this form of short-limbed dwarfism, hydrops is usually present, the chest is extremely narrow due to the very short horizontal ribs, and the long bones are extremely short and jagged.

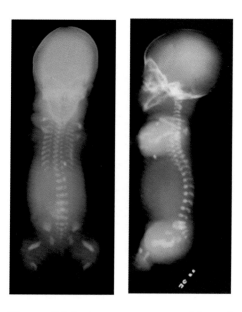

2.76

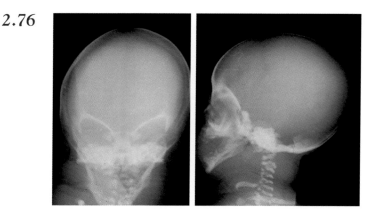

2.77

Figure 2.77. Skull radiograph, anteroposterior and lateral, showing the poor mineralization. Note the high clavicles.

Figure 2.76. Anteroposterior and lateral radiograph of another infant with Saldino-Noonan syndrome. Note the horizontal, very short ribs, the high clavicles and the extremely short, jagged long bones.

2.78

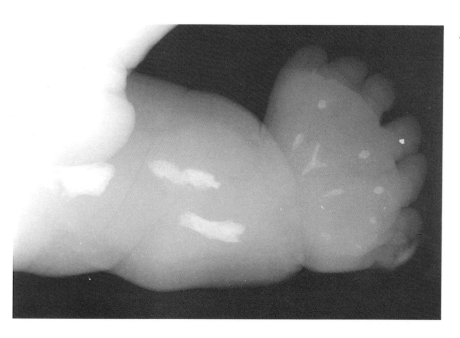

Figure 2.78. A close-up of the right upper extremity showing the extremely short, jagged long bones and poor development of the metacarpals and phalanges. Note the polydactyly.

2.79

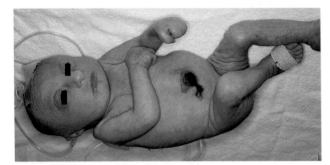

Figure 2.79. In Seckel's bird-headed dwarfism there is severe growth retardation with proportional dwarfism. This infant at 35 weeks gestation had a birth weight of 910 g, a length of 31.5 cm, and a head circumference of 23 cm, all less than the 10th percentile. There was severe microcephaly with premature fusion of all sutures, prominent eyes, a prominent beak-like nose, micrognathia, and malformed ears (low-set and lack of lobe). These infants have postnatal growth retardation and moderate to severe mental retardation.

2.80

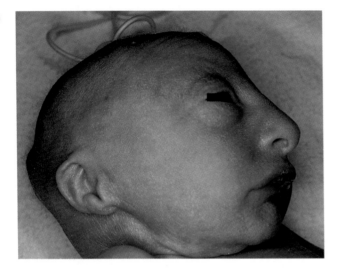

Figure 2.80. A close-up of the face of the same infant showing the severe microcephaly, the prominent eyes, the beak-like nose, and micrognathia. Note the low-set ear with lack of ear lobe. On CT scan the ventricles were barely perceptible and small in size.

2.81

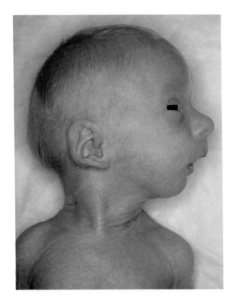

Figure 2.81. A less severe example of the Seckel's bird-headed dwarfism in which the microcephaly is striking but the other features are not as prominent.

2.82

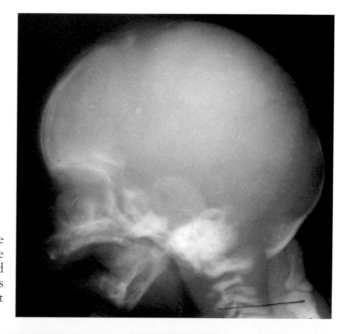

Figure 2.82. Radiograph of the skull in the same infant with Seckel's bird-headed dwarfism. Note the narrow (but not closed) sutures and tooth bud mineralization (incisors and first molars) in this infant. The tooth mineralization indicates that this infant had a gestational age of 35 weeks.

Figure 2.83. This infant is a typical example of spondylothoracic dysplasia (Jarcho-Levin syndrome). She had marked shortness of the neck and posterior aspect of the chest, with an increased diameter of the thoracic cage. The limbs were long and thin with tapering digits. Note the broad forehead and wide nasal bridge with anteverted nares. These infants typically have multiple anomalies of the vertebrae and a short thorax with a diminished number of ribs.

2.83

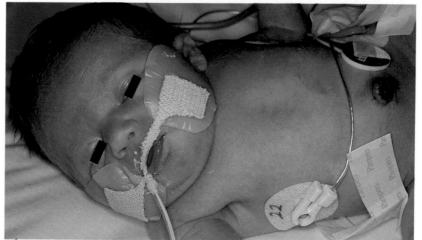

2.84

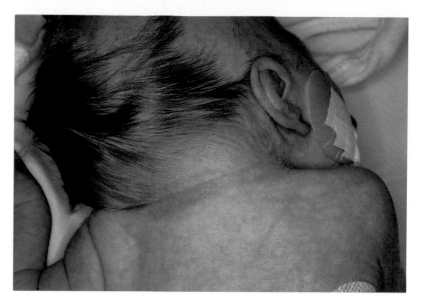

Figure 2.84. View of the back of the head and neck of the same infant showing the marked shortness of the neck and prominence of the occiput.

2.85

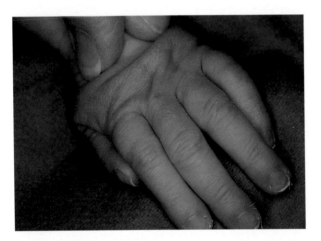

Figure 2.85. The fingers of the same infant as in Figure 2.83 and 2.84 show the typical long tapering digits (arachnodactyly) which are often noted in spondylothoracic dysplasia.

2.86

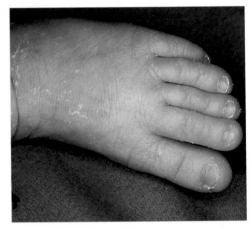

Figure 2.86. In this figure, note the extremely long tapering toes of the same infant.

2.87

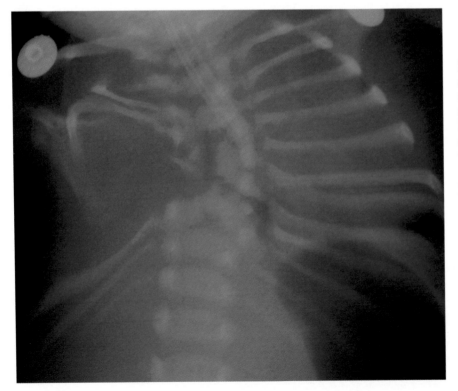

Figure 2.87. Chest radiograph of an infant with spondylothoracic dysplasia showing the grotesque and bizarre deformity of the ribs and spine. There is marked vertebral column shortening and numerous vertebral anomalies consisting of hemivertebrae, absent vertebrae, cleft vertebrae, and open neural arches. The severe deformity of the spinal column leads to posterior crowding and a fanlike appearance of the ribs on the frontal radiograms. The thorax is short on the right side due to a diminished number of ribs. The rib deformities are asymmetric.

2.88

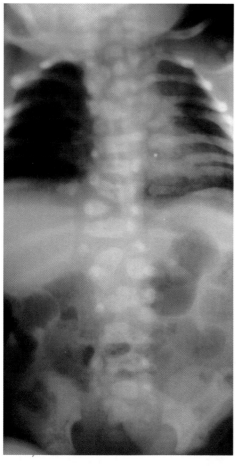

2.89

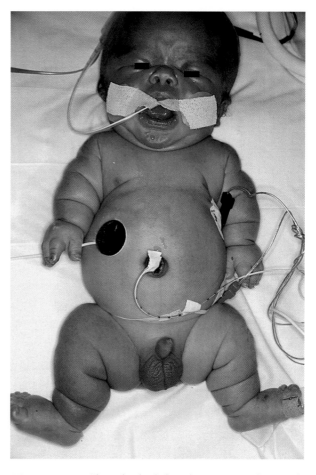

Figure 2.88. Radiograph of the thorax and abdomen in a less severe example of spondylothoracic dysplasia. Note the marked abnormalities in segmentation of the vertebrae. These abnormalities extend the total length of the spine, resulting in marked deformity of the spine (scoliosis, kyphosis).

Figure 2.89. Short-limbed dwarfism in an infant with thanatophoric dysplasia. This form of dwarfism is more common in males. Note the large head and hypertelorism. The chest is markedly narrowed with a large protruding abdomen. The limbs are short and there are increased skin folds about the extremities. These infants do not survive.

2.90

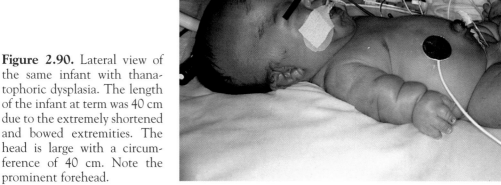

Figure 2.90. Lateral view of the same infant with thanatophoric dysplasia. The length of the infant at term was 40 cm due to the extremely shortened and bowed extremities. The head is large with a circumference of 40 cm. Note the prominent forehead.

2.91

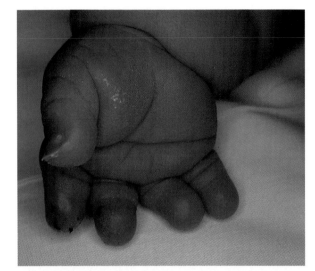

Figure 2.91. The right hand of the same infant demonstrating the marked brachydactyly and a single palmar crease.

2.92

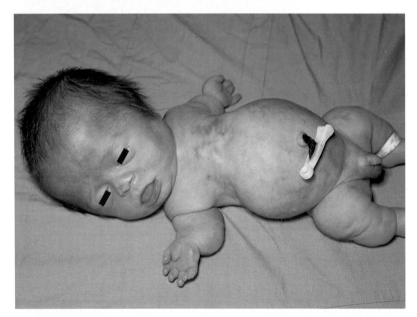

Figure 2.92. Another example of an infant with thanatophoric dysplasia. Note the hypotonia, large head, narrow thorax due to short ribs, prominent abdomen, and markedly shortened extremities. These infants with their large head and micromelia may be mistakenly diagnosed as having achondroplasia.

2.93

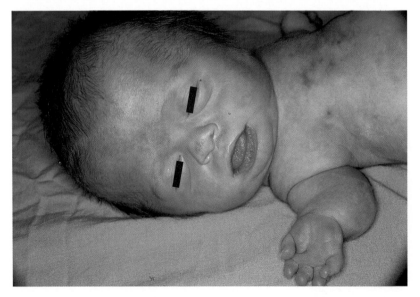

Figure 2.93. A close-up of the face of the same infant showing the large head, prominent forehead, hypertelorism, and flat nasal bridge. Note the narrow chest and short upper extremity with brachydactyly.

2.94

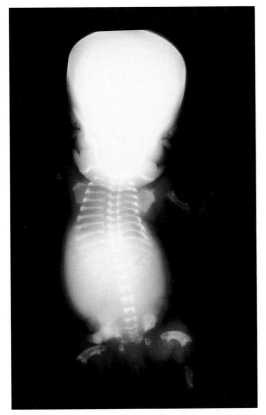

Figure 2.94. Body radiograph of an infant with thanatophoric dysplasia. Note the large head, narrow thorax due to short ribs, the typical V-shaped clavicles, and the prominent abdomen. Also note the marked flattening of the vertebral bodies. The ossification centers of the vertebrae are reduced.

2.95

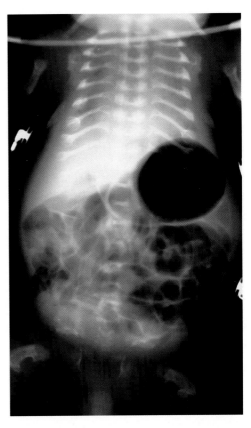

Figure 2.95. Anteroposterior radiograph of chest and abdomen in an infant with thanatophoric dysplasia. Note the short ribs which result in a narrow chest and the marked flattening of the vertebral bodies. The long bones demonstrate the marked shortening and bowing with the cupped irregular flaring of the proximal and distal metaphyses (the "telephone receiver" sign) which is especially noted in the femora.

2.96

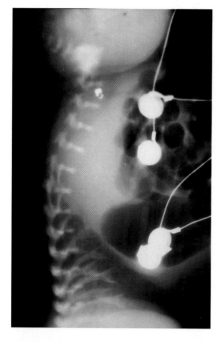

2.97

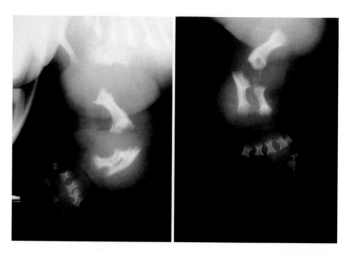

Figure 2.97. Radiograph of the upper extremities in an infant with thanatophoric dysplasia. Note the extremely shortened long bones with proximal and distal metaphyseal flaring.

Figure 2.96. Lateral radiograph of the same infant showing the marked flattening of the vertebral bodies and flat ends to the ribs. In an infant with short-limbed dwarfism, this finding is diagnostic of thanatophoric dysplasia.

2.98

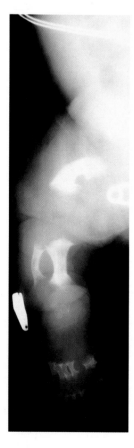

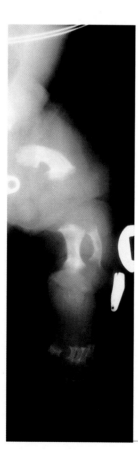

Figure 2.98. Radiograph of the lower extremities of the same infant again demonstrating the marked shortening of long bones with proximal and distal metaphyseal flaring.

Chapter 3
Non Chromosomal Syndromes, Associations, and Sequences

A syndrome, association, sequence, or complex is a constellation of abnormal physical signs, each nonspecific in isolation but resulting in a mosaic that can be diagnosed with confidence. The pathogenic mechanisms involved are variable. The clinical presentation depends on the pathogenic mechanism and the time of occurrence. Approximately 2% of all newborn infants have a significant malformation which may be relatively simple or complex. The later the defect develops in gestation, the more simple the malformation. In 10% of these infants, a chromosomal abnormality can be detected. In approximately 20%, the malformations are based on a single gene defect, with autosomal dominant disorders predominating. Multifactorial inheritance accounts for 30% of neonates with malformations. A small percentage of malformations is seen in infants born to diabetic mothers or mothers who have received a known teratogenic drug. The remaining 35% of newborn infants have no identifiable cause for their malformations. In infants with malformations, 7.5% are associated with deformations (see Volume I, Chapter 5). Malformations and deformations may recur with a similar pattern. Disruptions tend to be sporadic and no two cases are exactly alike. Due to limitations of space, this section can demonstrate only some very characteristic findings; therefore the clinician should not consider these descriptions to be complete and should refer to other references as needed.

3.1

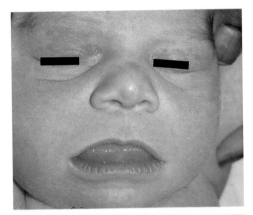

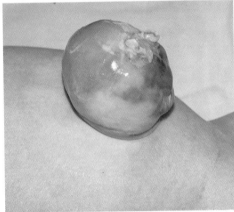

3.2

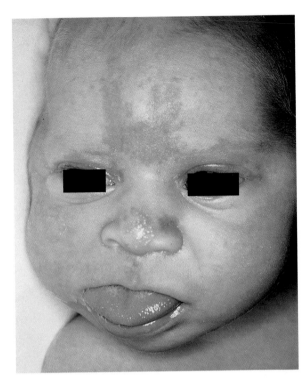

Figure 3.1. The top half of the figure shows macroglossia and a nevus flammeus; the lower portion shows an omphalocele; both in an infant with Beckwith-Wiedemann syndrome (*exomphalos-macroglossia-gigantism* [EMG] syndrome). It is usually sporadic and 60% of cases occur in females. Hemihypertrophy occurs in 10 to 15% of the infants.

Figure 3.2. Another example of an infant with the typical macrosomia (birthweight of 3950 g), polycythemia (hematocrit 66%) and hypoglycemia. Note the macroglossia, nevus flammeus over the glabellar region and the eyelids, and the prominent eyes with relative infraorbital hypoplasia.

3.3

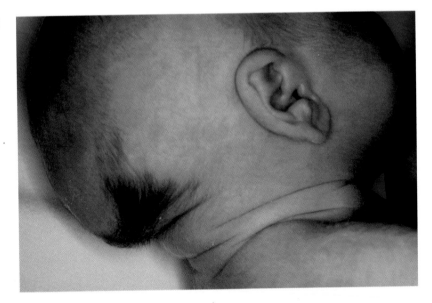

Figure 3.3. This infant with Beckwith-Wiedemann syndrome shows the prominent occiput and typical transverse crease in the lobe of the ear.

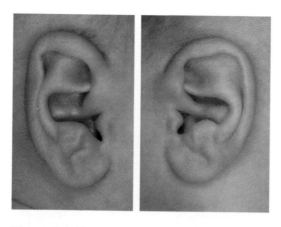

3.4

Figure 3.4. Transverse creases of the lobes of the ears in an infant with Beckwith-Wiedemann syndrome.

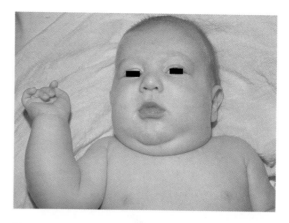

3.5

Figure 3.5. This 2-month-old infant with Caffey's syndrome (infantile cortical hyperostosis) shows the characteristic swelling of the jaw and right forearm. It usually occurs in a well-nourished infant. When the jaw is involved there is usually marked swelling of the face, mainly localized over the jaw. Most commonly this condition is diagnosed in the first few months of life, but congenital Caffey's syndrome has been reported.

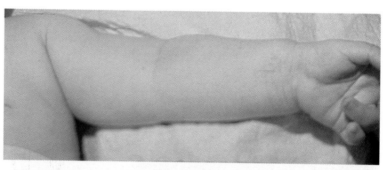

3.6

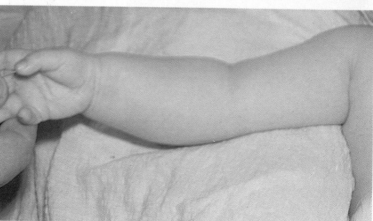

Figure 3.6. The same infant with Caffey's syndrome. Note that the left arm is normal but the right forearm is swollen and tender.

3.7

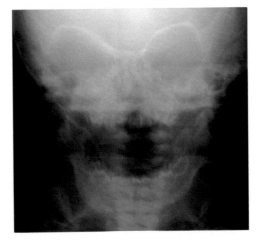

Figure 3.7. A radiograph showing the cortical hyperostosis of the jaw in an infant at the age of 4½ months.

3.8

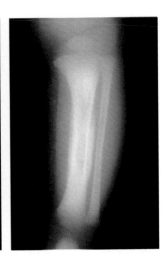

Figure 3.8. Lower extremity radiograph of the same infant at the age of 1 month. Note the early cortical hyperostosis of the femur and tibia.

3.9

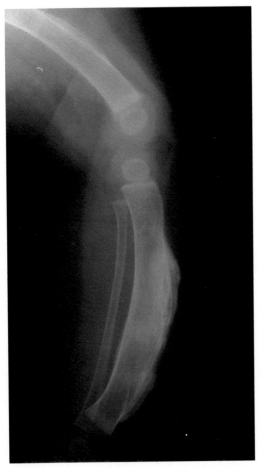

Figure 3.9. Follow-up radiograph of the lower extremity in the same infant at the age of 4½ months shows the marked cortical hyperostosis of the left tibia. Periosteal thickening of the long bones with translucent bands at the distal epiphyseal ends is diagnostic. Later, the bones expand and the cortex is thinned. The enlarged medullary cavity has little trabeculation and the soft tissue is swollen. The condition is self-limiting.

3.10

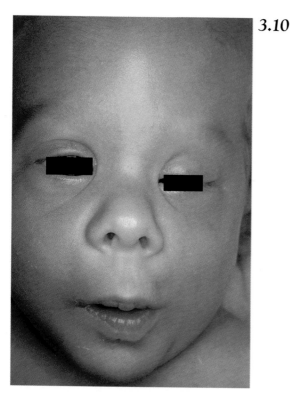

3.11

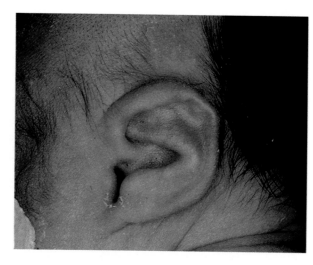

Figure 3.11. Abnormal ear in an infant with the CHARGE association.

Figure 3.10. Infant with the CHARGE association. Occurrence is non-random and is characterized by *c*oloboma, *h*eart disease, *a*tresia of the choanae, *r*etarded postnatal *g*rowth and development, genitourinary anomalies, and *e*ar anomalies and deafness. Most infants have some degree of mental deficiency. The coloboma commonly involves the retina but may range in severity from an isolated coloboma of the iris to anophthalmos.

3.12

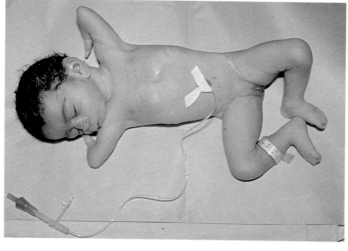

Figure 3.12. Cornelia de Lange's syndrome (Brachmann-de Lange syndrome: typus degenerativus amstelodamensis). One hundred percent of these infants have shortness of stature of prenatal onset, mental retardation and sluggish physical activity, hypoplastic nipples, initial hypertonicity and a low-pitched, weak, growling cry in infancy. Most of the infants have early feeding difficulties and early growth failure. In this infant note the bushy eyebrows and micromelia.

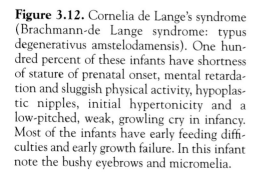

3.13

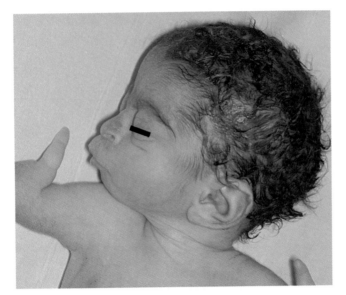

Figure 3.13. Close-up of face of the same infant as in Figure 3.12. Note the hirsutism, bushy eyebrows, downward slanting palpebral fissures, and micrognathia.

3.14

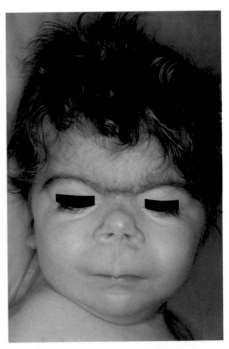

Figure 3.14. This infant with Cornelia de Lange's syndrome shows many of the characteristic findings: coarse, mop-like hair; bushy eyebrows and synophrys (confluent, thick eyebrows); long curly eyelashes; short nose with small anteverted nostrils; thin lips with a small midline beak of the upper lip; long philtrum; and downward curving of the angles of the mouth. The infants often have a mask-like expression.

3.15

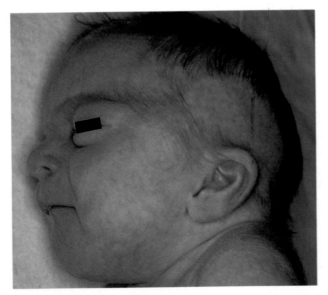

Figure 3.15. Another infant with Cornelia de Lange's syndrome showing the typical microbrachycephaly seen in over 90% of these infants, bushy eyebrows, small nose and micrognathia. Note the low-set ear and cutis marmorata which are also very common findings in Cornelia de Lange's syndrome.

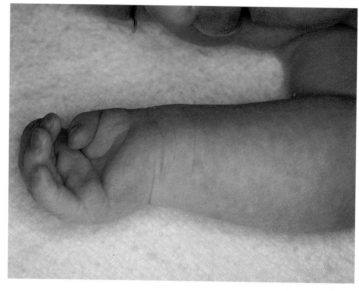

3.16

Figure 3.16. Anomalies of the extremities are common in infants with Cornelia de Lange's syndrome varying from the most severe (micromelia) to small hands and feet (microcheiria and micropodia). This infant with Cornelia de Lange's syndrome has microcheiria of the right hand. Both a single palmar crease (simian crease) and clinodactyly are very common in infants with this syndrome.

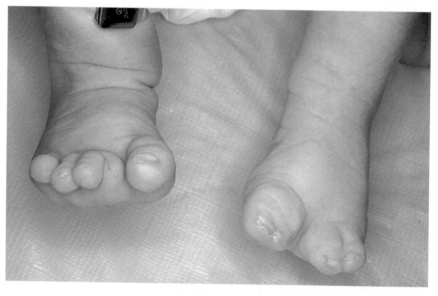

3.17

Figure 3.17. Syndactyly of the first, second, third and fourth toes in an infant with Cornelia de Lange's syndrome. The most common type of syndactyly is that of the second and third toes which is seen in many normal infants and in many syndromes.

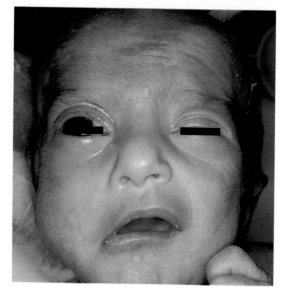

3.18

Figure 3.18. DiGeorge malformation complex. This is a primary defect of the fourth branchial arch and the third and fourth pharyngeal pouch. In this infant note the lateral displacement of the inner canthi (hypertelorism), the anteverted nares, and short philtrum with a cupid-bow mouth. This infant also had micrognathia, microcephaly, congenital heart disease (atrial septal defect and ventricular septal defect) and hypocalcemia. Note the congenital facial palsy which is not part of the complex. The EEG was grossly abnormal and the T cell count was decreased.

3.19

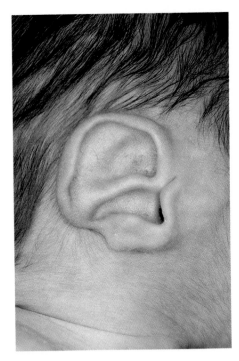

Figure 3.19. Abnormal dysplastic ear in the same infant. The acronym "CATCH 22 syndrome" has been applied to DiGeorge syndrome in that there are *c*ardiac defects, *a*bnormal facies, *t*hymic hypoplasia, *c*left palate, *h*ypocalcemia, and *22*q11 deletion.

3.20

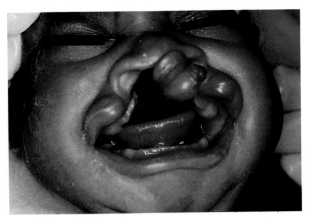

Figure 3.20. In the *ectrodactyly-ectodermal dysplasia-clefting* (EEC) syndrome there are varying manifestations of lobster-claw deformity (ectrodactyly) of the hands and feet and there is cleft lip/palate. The cleft lip is usually bilateral. Other manifestations include absence of the lacrimal puncta with tearing and blepharitis; abnormal teeth; malformations of the genitourinary (GU) tract such as cryptorchidism; and alterations in the skin and hair. Scalp hair, eyelashes and eyebrows are usually sparse and hair color is light. The nails may be hypoplastic and brittle. Most of these infants have normal intelligence. In this infant note the severe bilateral cleft lip and palate.

3.21

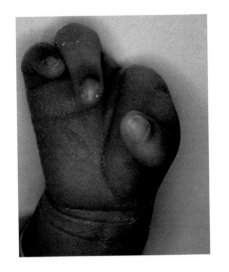
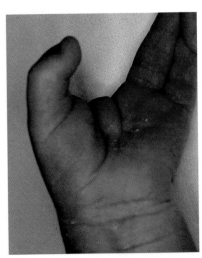

Figure 3.21. In this figure of the same infant note the ectrodactyly (lobster-clw deformity) of both hands. In this condition, usually all four extremities have a lobster-claw deformity.

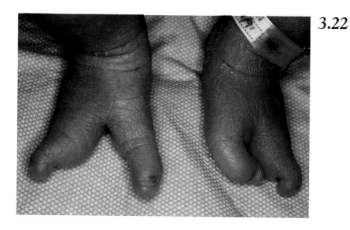

3.22

Figure 3.22. Dorsal view of the ectrodactyly of both feet of the same infant.

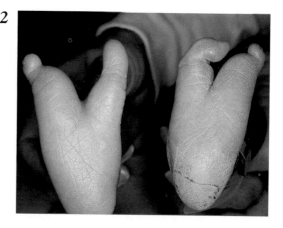

3.23

Figure 3.23. The same infant showing the soles of the feet.

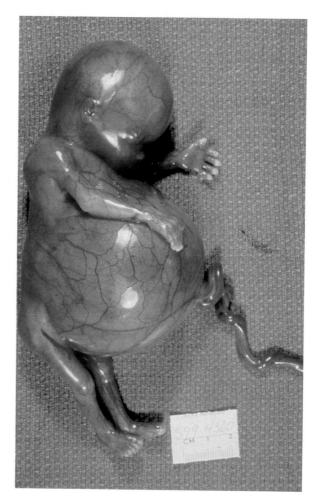

3.24

Figure 3.24. Eagle-Barrett syndrome (prune belly syndrome) is also described as the triad syndrome: absence of abdominal musculature, genitourinary tract abnormalities, and cryptorchidism. In this fetus there is a markedly distended abdomen due to a very distended bladder. It is now thought that the genitalia and urinary tract abnormalities are the precursor of the absence of abdominal musculature.

3.25

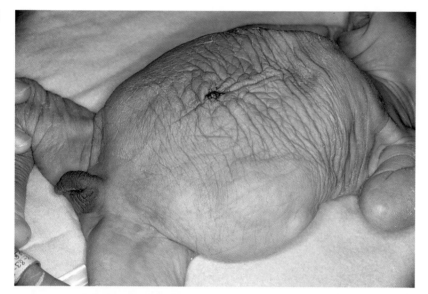

Figure 3.25. The characteristic findings of prune belly syndrome are present in this infant. Note the marked laxity of the abdominal wall giving it the appearance of a "prune," and the large mass on the left side of the abdomen due to massive dilatation of the ureter and hydronephrosis. Also note the cryptorchidism.

3.26

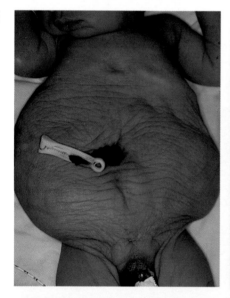 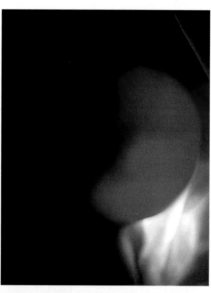

Figure 3.26. Another example of absence of abdominal musculature. Note the typical appearance of the prune belly on the left of the figure and the transillumination showing the massive hydroureter on the right.

3.27

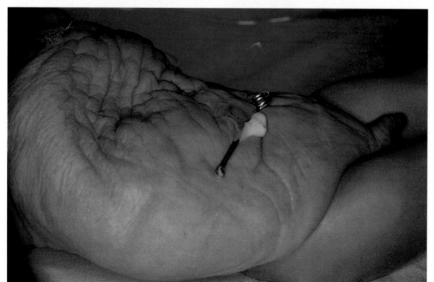

Figure 3.27. Appearance of absence of abdominal musculature in another infant.

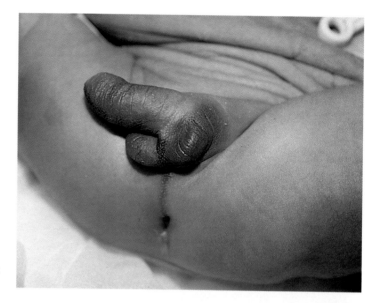

Figure 3.28. Cryptorchidism in an infant with prune belly syndrome.

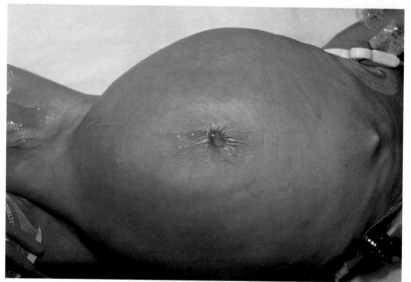

Figure 3.29. A common finding in infants with prune belly syndrome is a patent urachus.

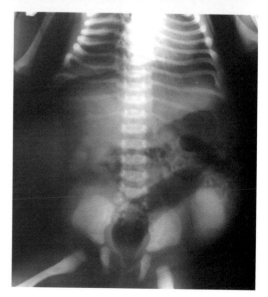

Figure 3.30. Radiograph of abdomen showing the bulging of the flanks and abnormal gas pattern due to genitourinary tract abnormalities in an infant with Eagle-Barrett syndrome.

3.31

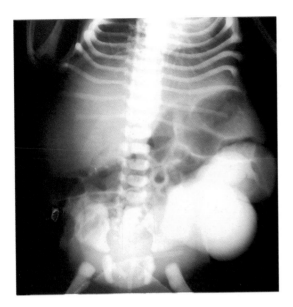

Figure 3.31. Contrast study in the same infant as in Figure 3.30 showing the massive hydroureter.

3.32

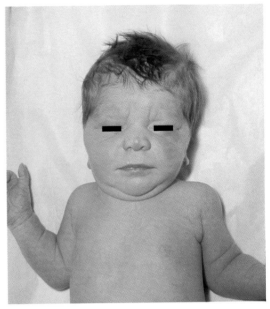

Figure 3.32. This infant with Ehlers-Danlos syndrome (cutis hyperelastica) presented at birth with marked hypotonia, joint hypermobility, and hyperextensibility of the skin. Note the epicanthal folds.

3.33

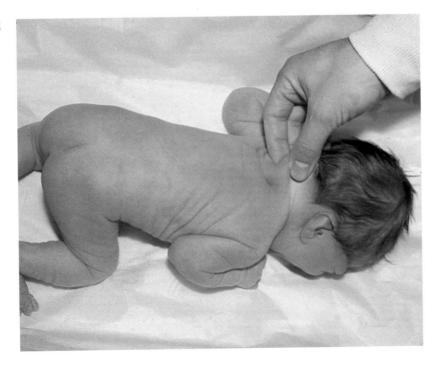

Figure 3.33. Figure of the same infant showing the webbing of the neck and hyperextensibility of the skin. The elasticity of the skin allows it to stretch and recoil, whereas in cutis laxa the skin hangs down in loose folds and does not recoil, and the joints are not hyperextensible as is seen in Ehlers-Danlos syndrome.

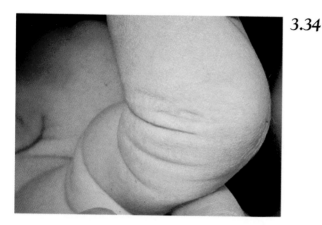

Figure 3.34. In the same infant note the hyperextensibility of the skin and the mild skin defects. There may be flat scars with paper-thin scar tissue, and hematomas occur after mild trauma in Ehlers-Danlos syndrome.

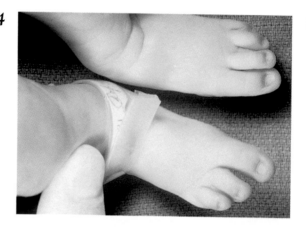

Figure 3.35. Other findings in Ehlers-Danlos syndrome include diaphragmatic hernia, congenital heart defects, and renal anomalies. There may be ectasia of portions of the gastrointestinal and respiratory tracts. The infant had an atrial septal defect, a small left diaphragmatic eventration, absence of the right mesocolon, and a double collecting system of the left kidney with an ectopic right kidney in the pelvis. The infant also demonstrates the second and fourth toes set dorsally to the first, third, and fifth toes and connected by a web.

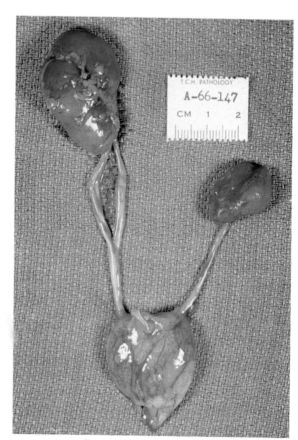

Figure 3.36. The renal system of the same infant at autopsy shows the ectopic right kidney which was in the pelvis and the left kidney with a double collecting system proximally.

3.37

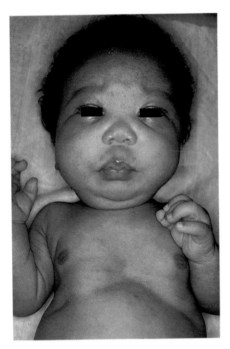

Figure 3.37. The fetal face syndrome (Robinow's syndrome or mesomelic dysplasia). These infants have slight to moderate shortness of stature, macrocephaly, a large anterior fontanelle, and frontal bossing with apparent hypertelorism, a short nose with anteverted nares, a long philtrum, and a small mouth with micrognathia. These result in a flat facial profile. The appearance of the face is similar to that of a fetus of about 8 weeks gestation. Hyperplastic alveolar ridges are present and a microphallus is a frequent finding.

3.38

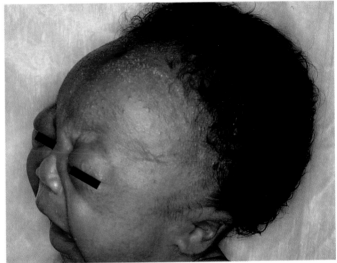

Figure 3.38. In this figure of the same infant note the marked frontal bossing, the large anterior fontanelle, the short nose, long philtrum, and micrognathia.

3.39

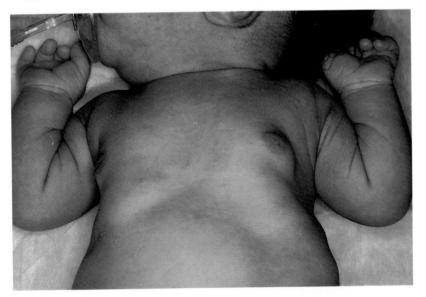

Figure 3.39. The chest and upper extremities of the same infant show the mesomelic dwarfism with the short forearms and brachydactyly. Mesomelic dwarfism affects the upper extremities more than the lower in these infants. There is mild pectus excavatum. Also note that this infant has some breast hypertrophy due to mastitis neonatorum.

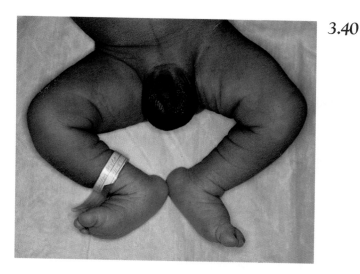

3.40

Figure 3.40. Note that the lower extremities of the same infant are normal except for the presence of bilateral rocker-bottom feet.

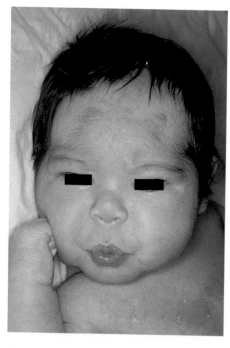

3.41

Figure 3.41. Infants with the femoral hypoplasia-unusual facies syndrome present with small stature and a typical facies. There are upslanting palpebral fissures, a short nose with hypoplastic alae nasi, a long philtrum, and a thin upper lip. A cleft palate may be present.

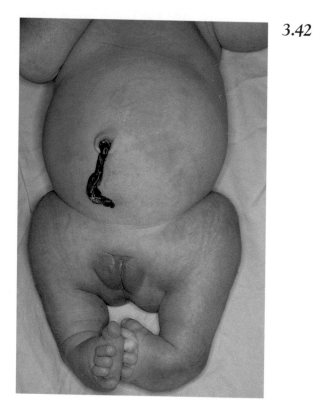

3.42

Figure 3.42. In this figure of the same infant note the abnormal lower extremities. These may be due to hypoplastic or absent femora and fibulae. In this infant the femora were absent and note also the bilateral talipes equinovarus. Hypoplasia of the humeri with restricted elbow movement may also occur in this syndrome.

3.43

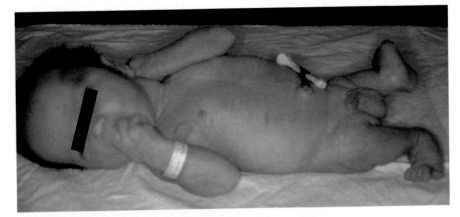

Figure 3.43. Another infant with the femoral hypoplasia-unusual facies syndrome. Note the small stature, predominantly the result of the small lower limbs.

3.44

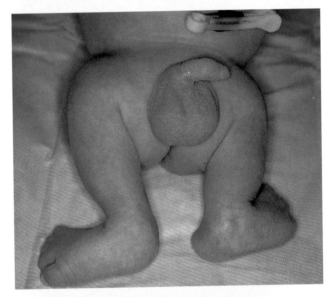

Figure 3.44. Close-up of the lower extremities of the same infant showing the absence of the femora.

3.45

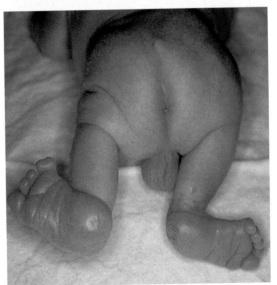

Figure 3.45. Posterior view of the lower extremities of the same infant.

3.46

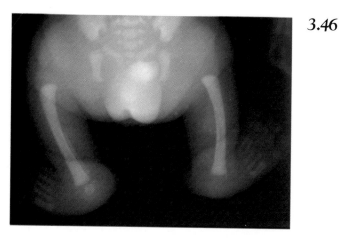

Figure 3.46. Radiograph of the lower extremities of the same infant showing the absence of femora bilaterally, a hypoplastic fibula on the right and an absent fibula on the left. In these infants, the acetabula may be hypoplastic and there may be a constricted iliac base with a vertical ischial axis.

3.47

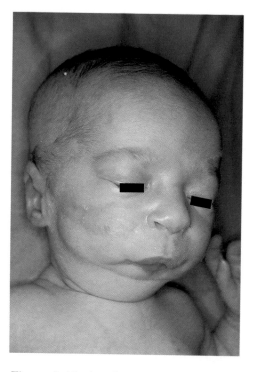

Figure 3.47. Another case of the femoral hypoplasia-unusual facies syndrome. Note the typical appearance of the face with the upslanting palpebral fissures, the short nose with hypoplastic alae nasi, long philtrum and micrognathia which was due to marked hypoplasia of the mandible. This infant also had a cleft palate which may be a part of this syndrome.

3.48

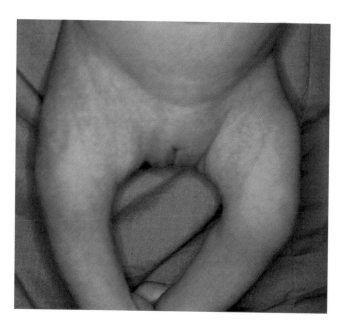

Figure 3.48. This figure of the same infant shows the short lower extremities with abnormal hypoplastic femora.

3.49

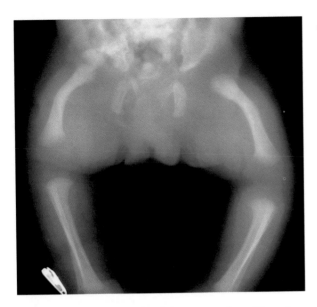

Figure 3.49. Radiograph of the same infant. The wings of the ilia are slenderized, the acetabular cavities are very shallow and ill formed, and there is bilateral dislocation of the hips. There are symmetric angular deformities in the midshafts of both femora which are shortened in length.

3.50

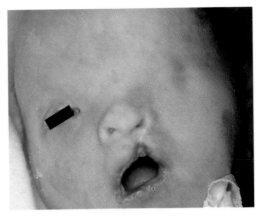

Figure 3.50. This infant, born at 35 weeks gestation, had Fraser's syndrome (cryptophthalmos syndrome). Note the cryptophthalmos on the left and the microphthalmia on the right. The infant had a cleft lip on the left and a high arched palate. There was subglottic tracheal obstruction. In Fraser's syndrome there is cryptophthalmos usually with a defect of the eye, and hair growth on the lateral forehead extends to the lateral eyebrow. Cryptophthalmos is bilateral in 50% of cases. There may be hypoplastic, notched nares and a broad nose with a depressed bridge. There are ear anomalies, most commonly cupping. Other findings in the syndrome include laryngeal stenosis or atresia, renal agenesis, and incomplete development of the male or female genitalia. There may be partial cutaneous syndactyly.

3.51

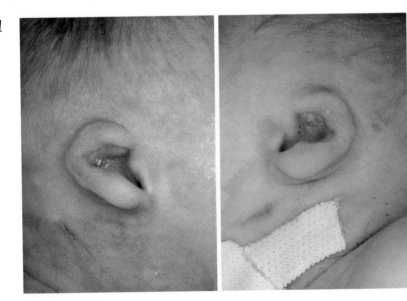

Figure 3.51. In this figure of the same infant, note the abnormal ears with marked cupping.

3.52

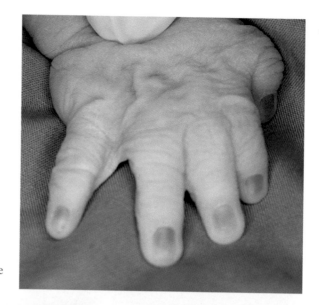

Figure 3.52. Cutaneous syndactyly (webbing) of the fingers is present in the same infant.

3.53

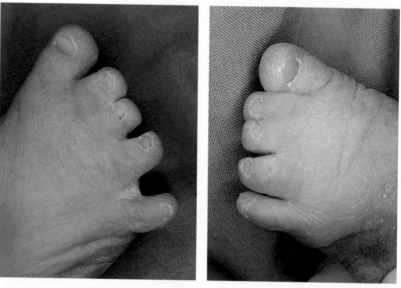

Figure 3.53. The same infant with Fraser's syndrome showing the webbing of the toes.

3.54

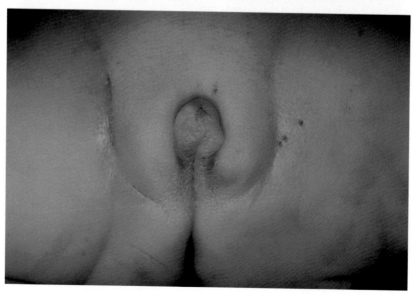

Figure 3.54. Clitoromegaly in the same infant with Fraser's syndrome. The uterus and ovaries were present on ultrasound and there was bilateral renal agenesis.

3.55

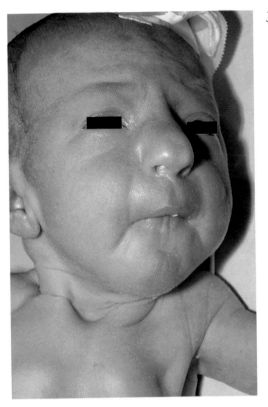

3.56

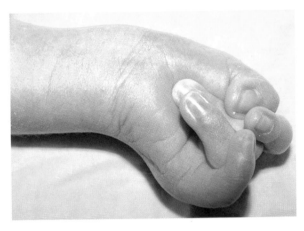

Figure 3.56. The upper extremity of the same infant with the Freeman-Sheldon syndrome. Note the ulnar deviation of the hand and contracted fingers.

Figure 3.55. Freeman-Sheldon syndrome ("whistling face" syndrome or cranio-carpotarsal dystrophy) is an autosomal dominant condition. Note the full forehead and mask-like facies with a small mouth giving a "whistling face" appearance. There is a broad nasal bridge with deep set eyes and blepharophimosis. The nose is small with hypoplastic alae nasi and a long philtrum. Note the H-shaped cutaneous dimpling on the chin and there may be a high palate and small tongue. These infants may have failure to thrive due to swallowing difficulties, but intelligence is in the normal range.

3.57

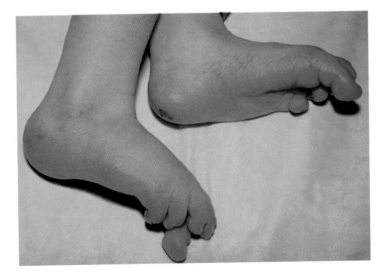

Figure 3.57. In this figure of the same infant, note the contractures of the toes. Talipes equinovarus may be present.

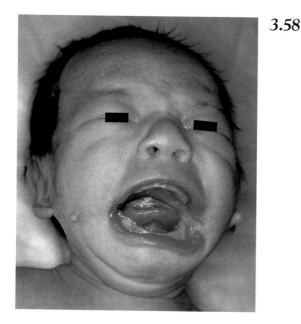

3.58

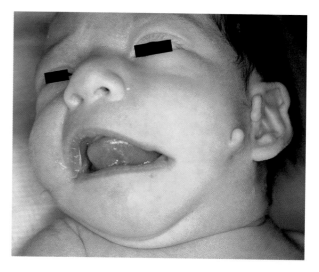

3.59

Figure 3.58. Goldenhar's syndrome (facio-auriculovertebral spectrum; oculoauriculovertebral dysplasia) is associated with abnormalities of the first and second branchial arches. This infant shows the antimongoloid slant, bilateral macrostomia, and skin tags. Over 90% of these infants have ear abnormalities (small or unusually shaped ears, preauricular tags, and pits). They may have abnormalities of the cervical vertebrae, particularly hemivertebra, coloboma of the upper eyelids, and epibulbar dermoids. Congenital heart disease may be present in one-third of these infants. More than 80% of the infants have normal intelligence.

Figure 3.59. Another infant with Goldenhar's syndrome showing the abnormal ear and preauricular skin tags in a line extending from the ear to the macrostomic mouth. Characteristic of Goldenhar's syndrome is the combination of unilateral facial hypoplasia, epibulbar dermoid, ocular abnormalities, preauricular appendages, and unilateral dysplasia of the auricle.

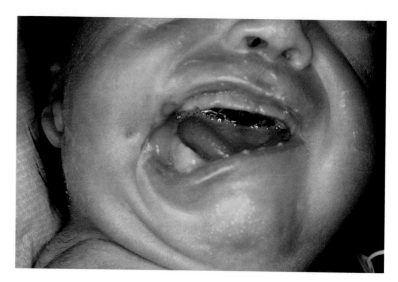

3.60

Figure 3.60. This infant is another example of Goldenhar's syndrome. She has macrostomia with a unilateral right facial cleft. In addition, there were ear epibulbar dermoids, and cardiac and vertebral abnormalities.

3.61

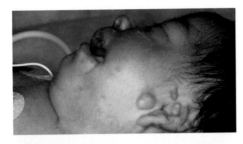

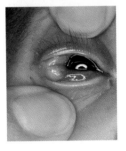
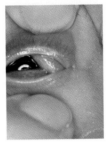

Figure 3.61. This composite figure of the same infant as in Figure 3.60 shows the abnormalities of the ears with preauricular tags and epibulbar dermoids.

3.62

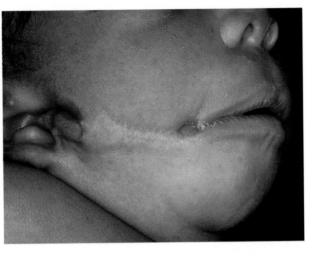

Figure 3.62. Another infant with Goldenhar's syndrome showing the lateral facial cleft, abnormal ear, preauricular skin tag, and abnormal skin from the corner of the mouth to the ear due to lack of normal fusion during development of the face.

3.63

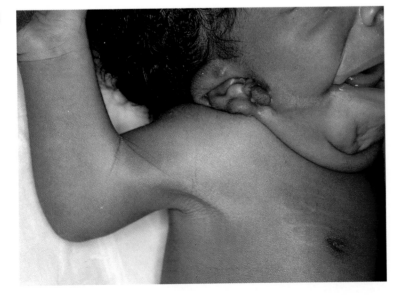

Figure 3.63. The same infant showing arthrogryposis.

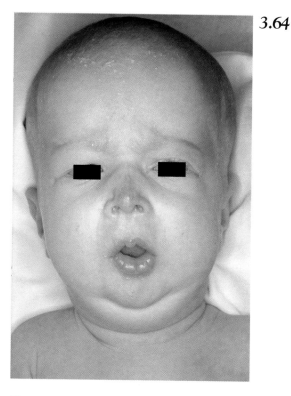

3.64

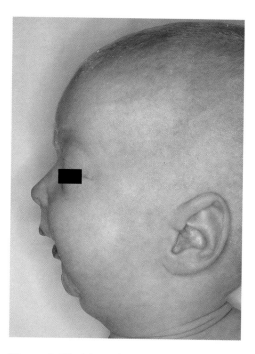

3.65

Figure 3.65. A lateral view of the same infant. Note the brachycephalic skull, small nose, micrognathia, and marked hypotrichosis. These infants have normal intelligence.

Figure 3.64. Infants with Hallermann-Streiff syndrome (oculomandibulofacial syndrome, François dyscephaly) have proportionate dwarfism. They also have brachycephaly with frontal and parietal bossing; hypotrichosis is present and the face appears small in relation to the skull. An antimongoloid slant of the eyes is common, and there is a narrow beaked nose and a hypoplastic mandible which gives the face a somewhat bird-like appearance. The mouth is small and there may be natal or supernumerary teeth. These infants often have bilateral congenital cataracts.

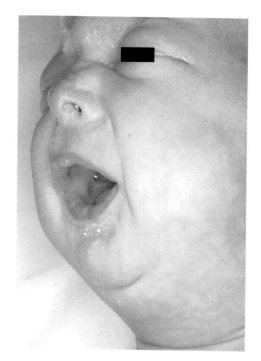

3.66

Figure 3.66. In this figure note the antimongoloid slant of the eyes, narrow beaked nose, small pinched mouth, micrognathia, hypoplastic mandible and hypotrichosis.

3.67

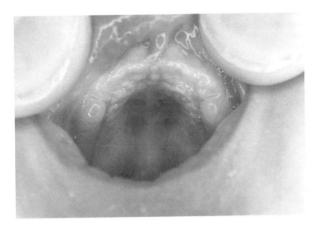

Figure 3.67. In this figure of the same infant as in Figure 3.66 note the high arched palate.

3.68

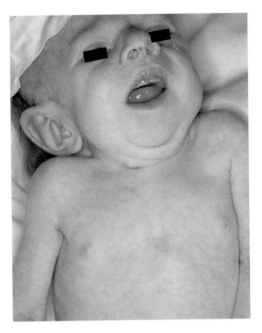

Figure 3.68. Infants with the Klippel-Feil syndrome or anomaly have a head which appears to be directly on the thorax. The facies is distorted and the ears are low set. Fusion or malformation of the cervical and upper thoracic vertebrae produces the short neck with head tilt and low posterior hairline. Strabismus is common.

3.69

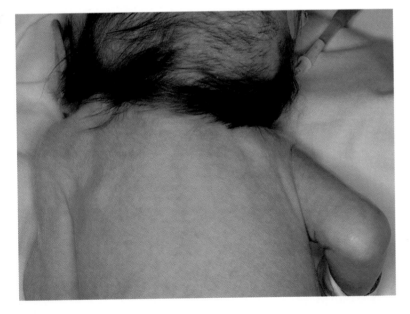

Figure 3.69. Posterior view of the same infant showing the short neck (congenital brevicollis) and the low hairline.

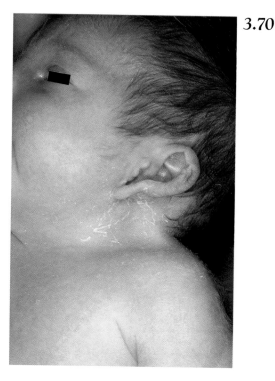

3.70

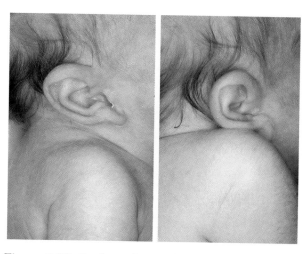

3.71

Figure 3.71. In this infant with the Klippel-Feil syndrome note the abnormal ear and short neck on the left. On the right, note that the abnormality of the ear results from pressure of the shoulder on the developing ear — a deformation.

Figure 3.70. A lateral view of the face, neck and chest of another infant with Klippel-Feil syndrome. Note the extremely short neck with low hairline and very abnormal ear.

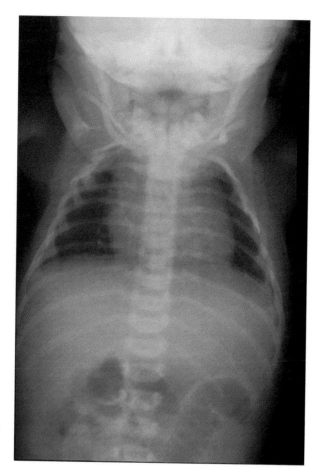

3.72

Figure 3.72. Anteroposterior radiograph of an infant with Klippel-Feil syndrome showing the numerous cervical spine vertebral body anomalies.

3.73

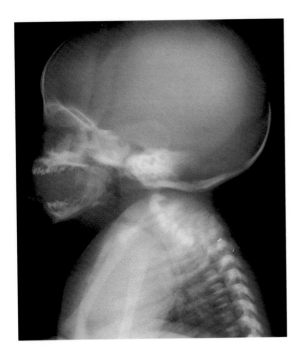

Figure 3.73. Lateral radiograph of the same infant as in Figure 3.72 with Klippel-Feil syndrome again shows cervical vertebrael anomalies resulting from abnormal fusion of the cervical vertebrae. There may be other associated skeletal defects such as the Sprengel's deformity or thoracic hemivertebrae. If the brachial plexus is involved, it may result in deformities of the hand.

3.74

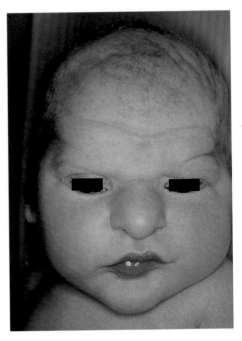

Figure 3.74. Infants with the Langer-Giedion syndrome have a bulbous nose, tented alae nasi, and a prominent elongated philtrum. There is a thin upper lip with mild micrognathia and mild microcephaly. Scalp hair is sparse. The ears are hypertrophic with excessive folding and tissue mass. The skin is redundant and loose. This infant, in addition to the above findings, had cutis verticis gyrata.

3.75

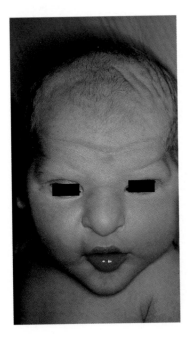 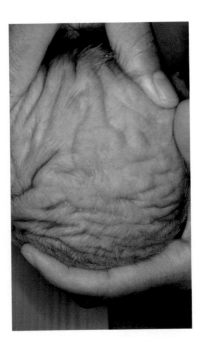

Figure 3.75. In this figure of the same infant again note the bulbous nose, thin upper lip on the left and the cutis verticis gyrata on the right. The trichorhinophalangeal syndrome has many similarities to Langer-Giedion syndrome except that the redundant skin and microcephaly are not present.

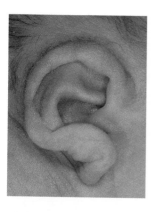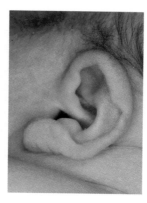

3.76

Figure 3.76. Close-up of the ears of the same infant showing the hypertrophy with excessive folding and tissue mass.

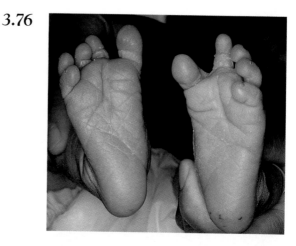

3.77

Figure 3.77. The same infant had large vertical creases on both plantar surfaces anteriorly. These are strongly associated with trisomy 8. The Langer-Giedion syndrome recently has been associated with a deletion of the long arm of chromosome 8.

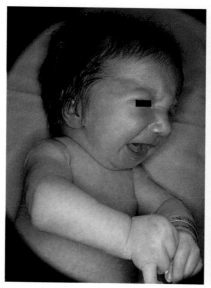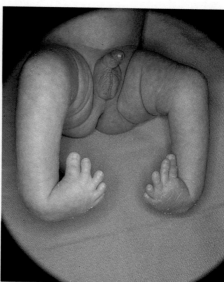

3.78

Figure 3.78. This infant with Larsen's syndrome demonstrates the prominent forehead, depressed nasal bridge, and dislocation of the elbows on the left. On the right there is dislocation of the hips, knees, and talipes equinovarus.

3.79

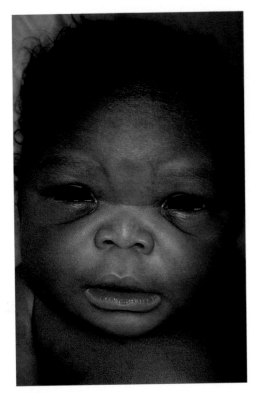

Figure 3.79. In Larsen's syndrome there is a flat facies associated with a prominent forehead, a flat and depressed nasal bridge, and the eyes are wide set.

3.80

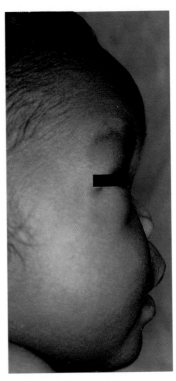

Figure 3.80. A lateral view of the face of the same infant shows the very flat facies associated with a prominent forehead and depressed nasal bridge. Note that the eyes are rather deep set.

3.81

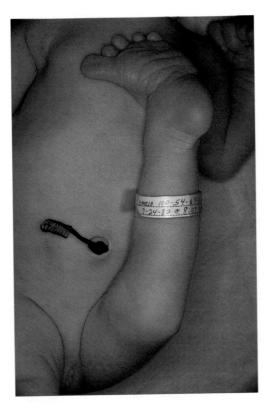

Figure 3.81. In this infant with Larsen's syndrome note the congenital dislocation of the left knee, metatarsus varus, and large big toe.

3.82

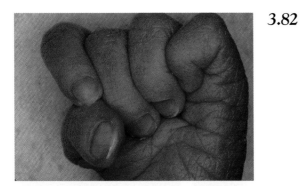

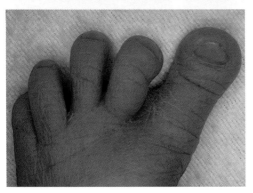

3.83

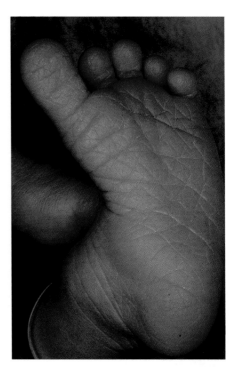

Figure 3.82. Infants with Larsen's syndrome have other characteristic findings in addition to the flat facies and multiple joint dislocations (elbows, hips, and knees). Note the broad spatulate thumb and altered hand position due to the short metacarpals (upper photo), and the big toe and hypoplastic nails (lower photo).

Figure 3.83. In the same infant, note the typical large big toe and metatarsus varus.

3.84

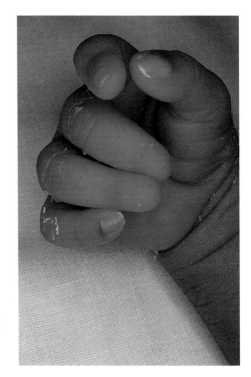

Figure 3.84. This infant with Larsen's syndrome has spatulate thumbs and shortened metacarpals. Also note the absence of nails on the third and fourth fingers of the right hand.

3.   3.91

3.92

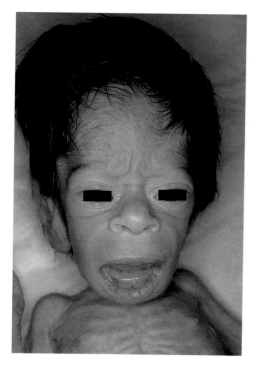

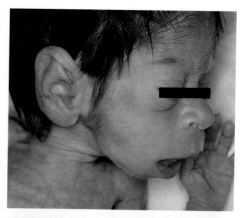

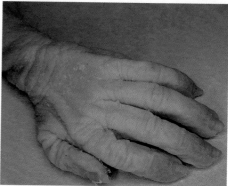

Figure 3.91. A close-up of the face of the same infant as in Figure 3.90 at the age of 3 weeks again shows the severe growth retardation, sunken cheeks, pointed chin, large mouth, large eyes that have a very alert expression, and large ears. Note the gingival hyperplasia.

3

Figure 3.92. A lateral view of the face of the same infant. Note the sunken face and very large ears in the upper half of the figure. The lower portion of the figure shows the large hands that are seen in these infants. Note the marked loss of subcutaneous tissue and wrinkled, loose skin. Infants with Donohue's syndrome commonly have large hands and feet. At autopsy the infant had cystic ovaries which are typically found in this condition.

3.93

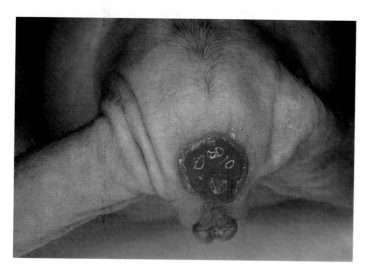

Figure 3.93. This infant, in addition, had a rectal prolapse. Note the wrinkled, loose skin associated with marked lack of adipose tissue.

3.94

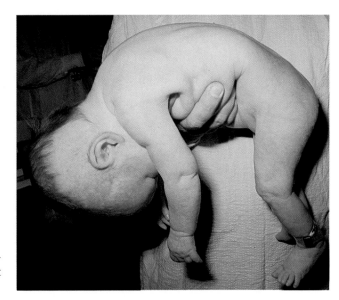

Figure 3.94. In Lowe syndrome (oculocerebrorenal syndrome) there is marked hypotonia and joint hypermobility.

3.95

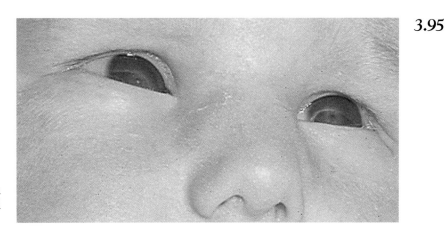

Figure 3.95. The same infant with Lowe syndrome has bilateral cataracts and epicanthic folds.

3.96

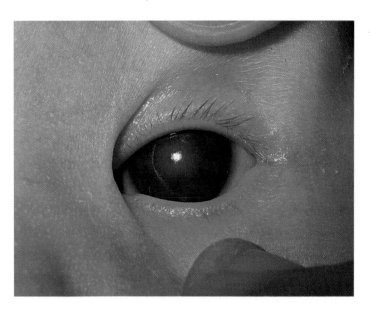

Figure 3.96. Corneal clouding and epicanthic folds are present in the same infant.

3.97

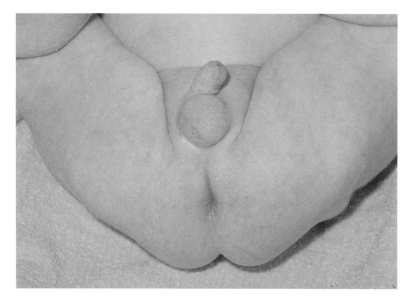

Figure 3.97. In Lowe syndrome, renal tubular dysfunction and cryptorchidism are common. Note the presence of cryptorchidism.

3.98

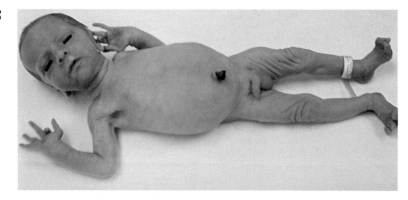

Figure 3.98. A term newborn with Marfan syndrome who had a birth weight of 3720 g and a length of 54 cm. Note the tall stature with long slim limbs and hypotonia. In Marfan syndrome, limbs are disproportionately long and trunk length is usually normal resulting in a low upper/lower segment ratio. Ophthalmologic and cardiovascular pathologies, such as dislocation of the lens and aneurysmal dilatation of the aorta, are usually noted after the neonatal period.

3.99

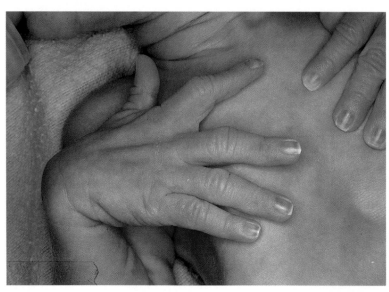

Figure 3.99. In this infant with Marfan syndrome, note the marked lengthening of the fingers (arachnodactyly). The diagnosis of Marfan syndrome may be difficult in the neonatal period because many normal infants appear to have long fingers. The combination of an increased birth length and a decreased upper / lower segment ratio should alert one to the possibility of this diagnosis. In older children the disproportion can often be detected by noting that the finger tips reach much further down the thigh than usual in the standing position.

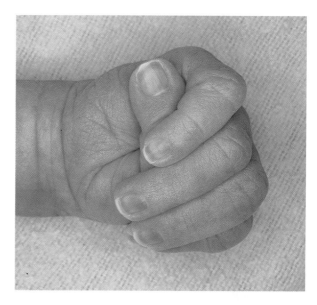

Figure 3.100. In Marfan syndrome when the patient makes a fist, the thumb often extends beyond the fifth finger as shown in the same infant.

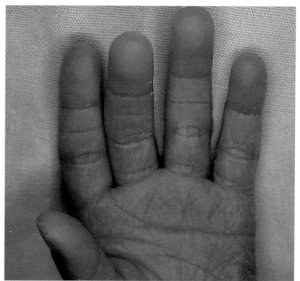

Figure 3.101. This neonate with Marfan syndrome exhibits the long fingers with increased creases on the fingers. This finding is common in infants who have increased mobility and hyperextensibility at the joints during development in utero and is seen in conditions such as Marfan syndrome and Larsen's syndrome.

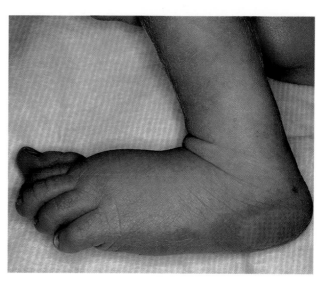

Figure 3.102. The same infant with Marfan syndrome shows the long foot and arachnodactyly.

3.103

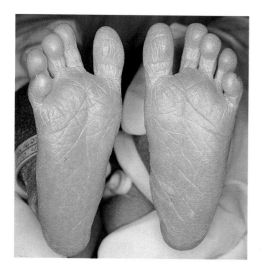

Figure 3.103. This is another example of long feet and toes in an infant with Marfan syndrome. Note the bilateral congenital curly toes. This infant had a birth length of 53 cm and an upper/lower segment ratio of 1.41. The normal upper/lower segment ratio at birth is 1.69 to 1.70. In short-limbed dwarfism and hypothyroidism it averages 1.8 or more, and in Marfan syndrome it averages 1.45.

3.104

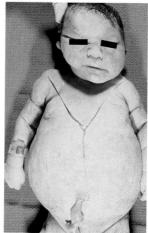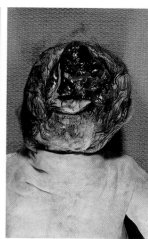

Figure 3.104. The typical findings in Meckel-Gruber syndrome (dysencephalia splanchnocystica) include encephalocele, polydactyly, and cystic dysplasia of the kidneys. In this infant there was marked oligohydramnios, deformations, encephalocele, hypoplastic lungs, infantile polycystic kidneys, and polydactyly. On the left note the marked abdominal distention due to the polycystic kidneys and on the right note the parieto-occipital encephalocele. (C. Langston)

3.105

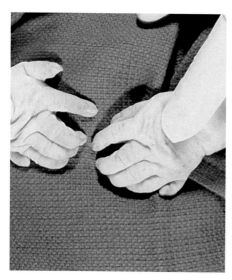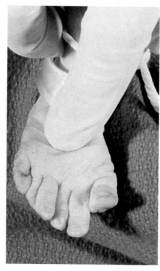

Figure 3.105. The same infant showing the polydactyly of both hands and polydactyly of the right foot. (C. Langston)

3.106

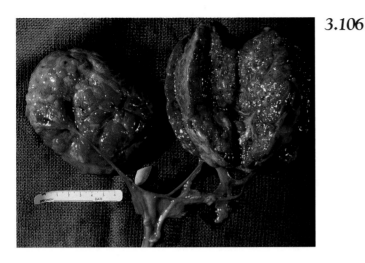

Figure 3.106. Bilateral infantile polycystic kidneys in the same infant with Meckel-Gruber syndrome. The right kidney weighed 210 g and the left kidney 200 g. (C. Langston)

3.107

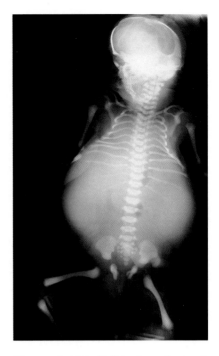

Figure 3.107. Full-body radiograph of the same infant. Note the marked skull defect associated with an encephalocele; the bell-shaped thorax and hypoplastic lungs; and the enlarged abdomen bulging in the flanks associated with the infantile polycystic kidneys.

3.108

Figure 3.108. This infant with Nager's acrofacial dysostosis syndrome shows the slight antimongoloid slant, prominent nose, malar hypoplasia, micrognathia, and atresia of the external auditory canal. Associated with the hypoplastic mandible may be a bony cleft of the mandibular symphysis. In addition, the infant had radial hypoplasia and absence of thumbs. This infant required an emergency tracheostomy. Also note the projection of the scalp hair onto the lateral cheek.

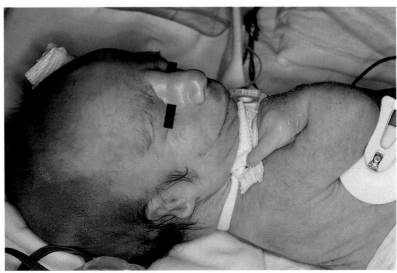

3.109

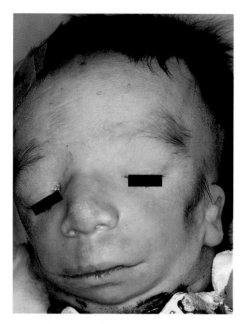

Figure 3.109. Frontal view of the face of the same infant as in Figure 3.108. The facial appearance resembles that of infants with Treacher-Collins syndrome. Note the partial absence of eyebrows which is another feature in these infants.

3.110

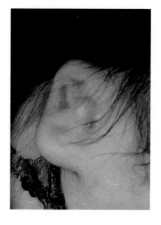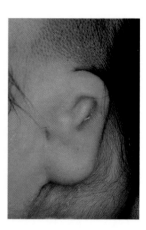

Figure 3.110. This figure shows the abnormal ears with atresia of the external auditory canals in the same infant.

3.111

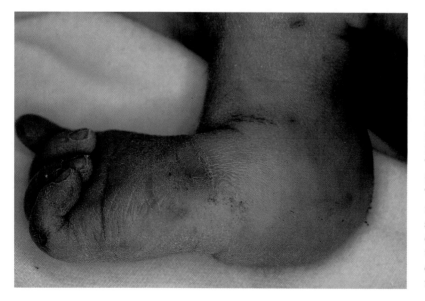

Figure 3.111. Hypoplastic radius and ulna and absent thumb in the right upper extremity of the same infant. Hypoplasia or aplasia of the radius and absence of the thumb may or may not be present in infants with Nager's syndrome. This infant also had these typical findings in both upper extremities. This results in short forearms and there may be proximal radioulnar synostosis and limitation of elbow extension. Postaxial hexadactyly of the hands and feet and synostosis of the metacarpals and metatarsals may occur.

3.112

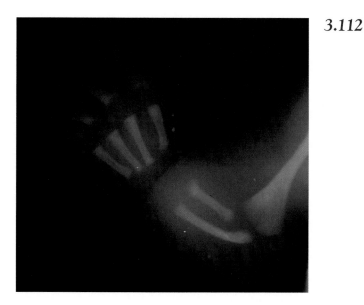

Figure 3.112. Radiograph of the right upper extremity showing the hypoplastic radius and ulna and absent right thumb.

3.113

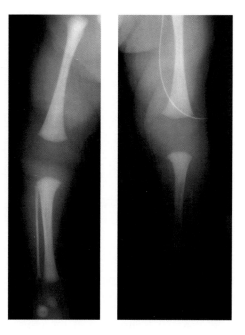

Figure 3.113. Radiograph of the lower extremities of the same infant showing hypoplasia of the right fibula and absence of the left fibula.

3.114

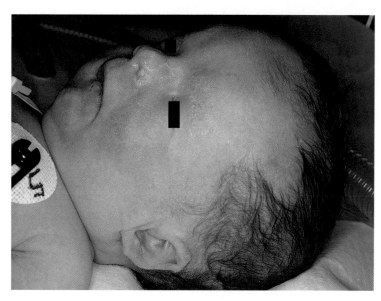

Figure 3.114. This infant with orofaciodigital syndrome type I (an X-linked dominant disorder limited to females because it is lethal in males) has an enlarged head from hydrocephalus.

3.115

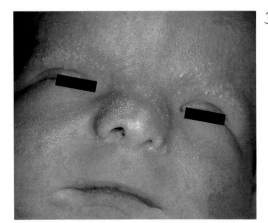

Figure 3.115. This frontal view of the same infant as in Figure 3.114 shows the typical facial appearance. Note the wide interorbital distance (euryopia), lateral displacement of the inner canthi, the flat midfacial region, and one nostril which is smaller than the other. The nasal root is broad, there is a short upper lip with a thin vermilion border, and typically milia are present in these infants.

3.116

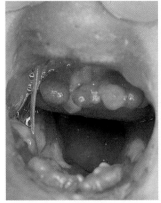
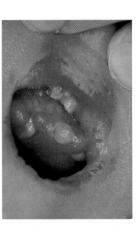

Figure 3.116. In these figures the same infant shows the clefting of the palate and the small hematomatous masses on the dorsal and ventral surfaces of the tongue. Neonatal teeth and ankyloglossia are present. There is also webbing between the buccal mucous membranes and the alveolar ridge.

3.117

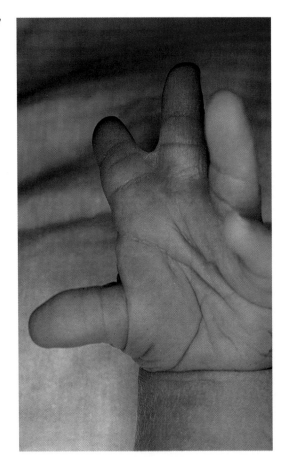

Figure 3.117. The same infant has brachydactyly, clinodactyly, and syndactyly of the fingers of the left hand.

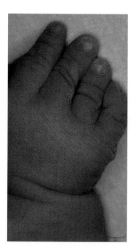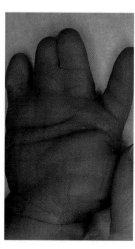

3.118

Figure 3.118. The right hand of the same infant with orofaciodigital syndrome again shows the brachydactyly and syndactyly on the right. Note the clinodactyly and prominence on the little finger due to postaxial polydactyly.

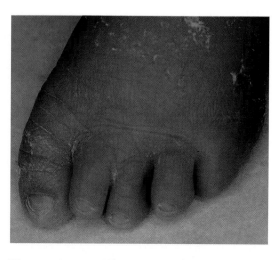

3.119

Figure 3.119. The same infant also shows marked brachydactyly of the toes. The hallux is inclined laterally and there is syndactyly of the second and third toes.

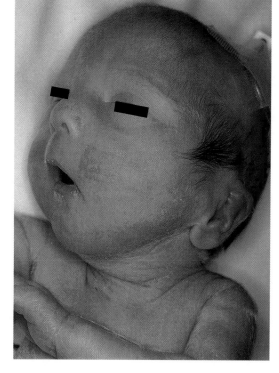

3.120

Figure 3.120. In the Pena-Shokeir phenotype type I (fetal akinesia/hypokinesia sequence), there is severe intrauterine growth retardation and diffuse atrophy of skeletal muscle resulting in arthrogryposis with the head circumference spared. There are low-set ears, a depressed tip of the nose, small mouth, and micrognathia. It is suggested that this phenotype is secondary to decreased in utero movement and as a result there is polyhydramnios (due to failure of normal swallowing) and a short umbilical cord. There may be severe neuromyopathic disease. Neuromuscular deficiency of the diaphragm and intercostal muscles results in pulmonary hypoplasia.

3.121

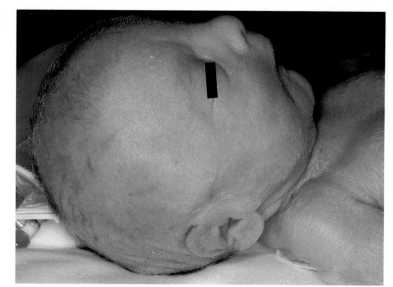

Figure 3.121. The lateral view of the same infant as in Figure 3.120 shows the poorly developed, low-set ear, depressed nasal tip, and micrognathia.

3.122

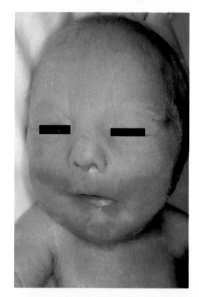

Figure 3.122. A close-up of the face of the same infant shows hypertelorism, telecanthus, and epicanthic folds, as well as the depressed nasal tip with a small mouth and micrognathia.

3.123

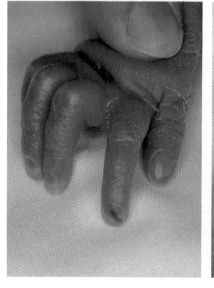
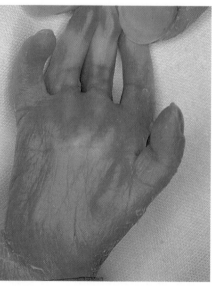

Figure 3.123. This same infant shows camptodactyly due to contractures in the fingers. Also note the poor dermal ridges and absence of flexion creases on the fingers and palms due to lack of fetal movement in the early weeks of gestation.

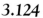

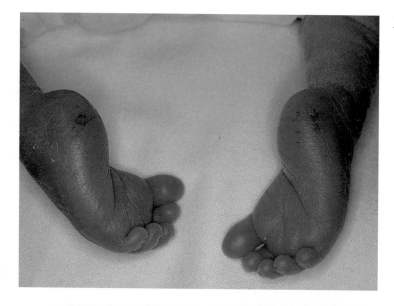

Figure 3.124. Talipes equinovarus in the same infant.

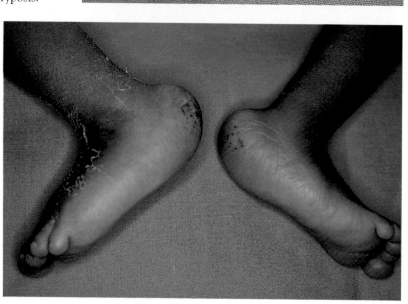

Figure 3.125. Another infant with the fetal akinesia sequence showing the marked lack of dermal ridges and creases. This infant had the typical dysmorphic features of the face, webbing of the neck, and severe intrauterine growth retardation with generalized arthrogryposis.

Figure 3.126. The same infant also had rocker-bottom feet.

3.127

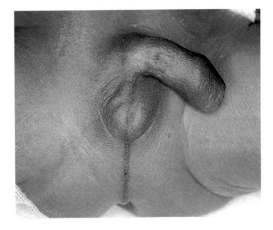

Figure 3.127. Cryptorchidism is common in infants with the fetal akinesia sequence.

3.128

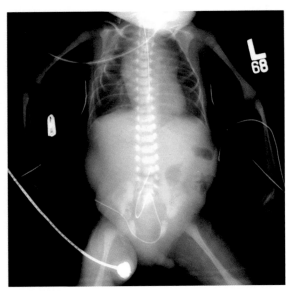

Figure 3.128. In a body radiograph of the same infant with the fetal akinesia sequence, note the thin gracile ribs, long thin clavicles, and thinning of all the long bones. The soft tissue in the extremities shows a lack of muscle mass. The appearance of the gracile ribs and long clavicles are also seen in trisomy 18 and myotonic dystrophy.

3.129

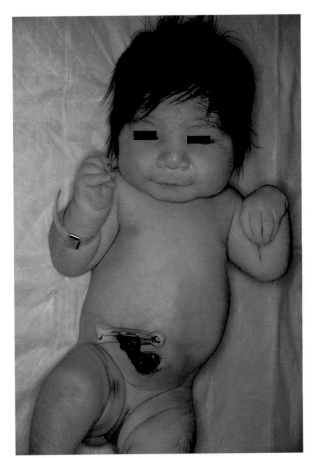

Figure 3.129. This infant with cerebrooculofacioskeletal (COFS) syndrome (Pena-Shokeir syndrome type II) presented with generalized hypotonia, hirsutism, characteristic facial features, widely spaced nipples, joint contractures, camptodactyly, and rocker-bottom feet.

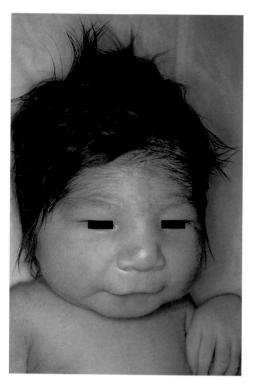

3.130

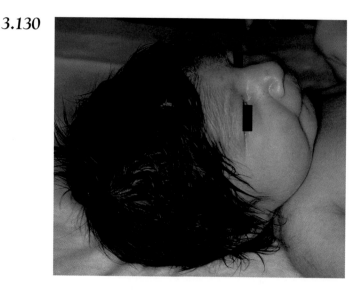

3.131

Figure 3.131. A lateral view of the head and face of the same infant shows the hirsutism, microcephaly, blepharophimosis, deep-set eyes, upper lip overlapping the lower lip, and micrognathia.

Figure 3.130. A close-up view of the face of the same infant showing the characteristic facial features. Note the hirsutism, deep-set eyes, prominent root of the nose, upper lip overlapping the lower lip, and micrognathia.

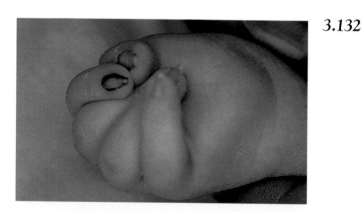

3.132

Figure 3.132. In the close-up of the hand of this infant with COFS syndrome in the upper figure note the camptodactyly, and in the lower figure with the hand open, note the absence of finger creases due to lack of fetal movement early in gestation.

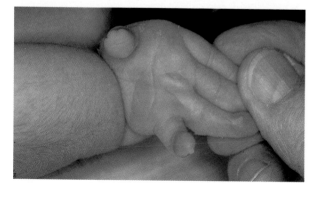

3.133

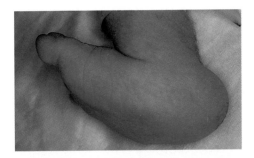

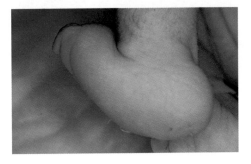

3.134

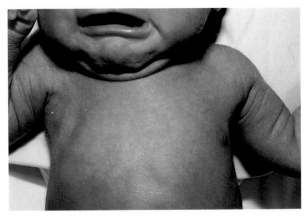

Figure 3.134. Infant with Poland's anomaly showing unilateral absence of the sternal and costal portions of the pectoralis major muscle and brachysyndactyly of the hand on the ipsilateral side. There may be absence or hypoplasia and upward displacement of the nipple and breast on the affected side.

Figure 3.133. The same infant as in Figure 3.132 demonstrates rocker-bottom feet. Note the marked contracture accompanying this as seen in the right foot in the lower figure. These infants also have a longitudinal groove in the soles along the second metatarsal.

3.135

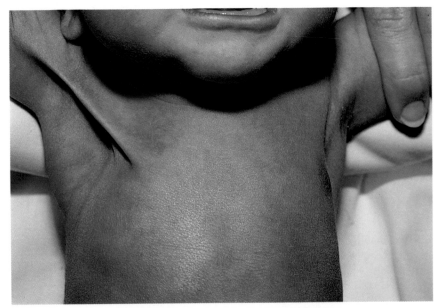

Figure 3.135. If the abnormality is not obvious, then extending the arms is a means of better demonstrating the abnormality as seen in the same infant. Note the absence of the nipple. Occasionally there may be some abnormalities underlying the defect.

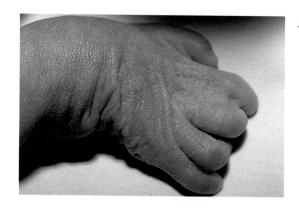

3.136

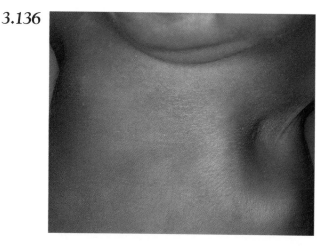

3.137

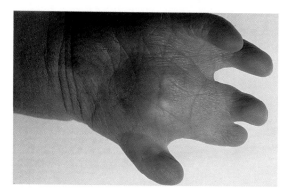

Figure 3.137. Another example of Poland's anomaly. In this infant the defect is more severe, in that in addition to the lack of the pectoralis major there are defects in other muscles such as the absence of the pectoralis minor. In Poland's anomaly, 75% of the infants are male and in 70% the right side is affected.

Figure 3.136. The hands of the same infant show the brachysyndactyly. The hand on the affected side is usually smaller than that on the unaffected side. There is usually no bony synostosis. Less commonly the forearm is smaller on the affected side.

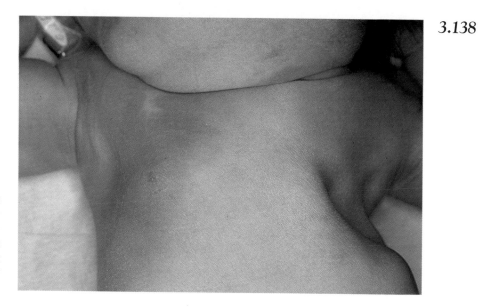

3.138

Figure 3.138. The defect the chest wall was due to a deformation resulting from the abnormal hand being held in the "position-of-comfort" where it was lodged during the last few weeks of gestation.

3.139

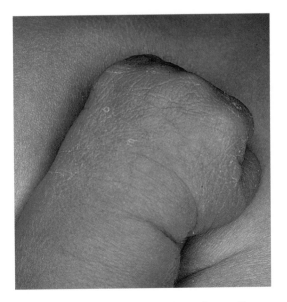

Figure 3.139. A close-up of the infant in Figure 3.138 showing the hand placed in the defect.

3.140

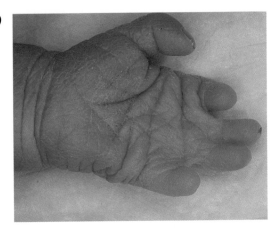

Figure 3.140. A close-up of the left hand showing the marked brachysyndactyly.

3.141

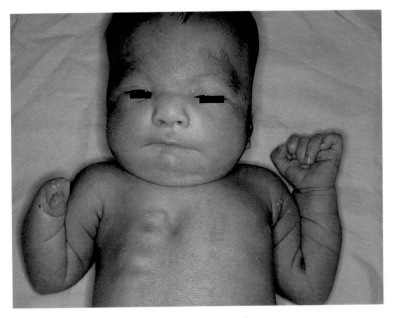

Figure 3.141. In about 15% of cases there is an association of Poland's anomaly with Möbius' syndrome. In Poland's anomaly the hand anomalies are usually unilateral, whereas in Möbius' syndrome they are usually bilateral. This infant with Poland's anomaly and Möbius' syndrome shows the mask-like facies, ptosis of eyelids, drooping of the angles of the mouth, and the absence of the right pectoralis with a hypoplastic right forearm and hand.

3.142

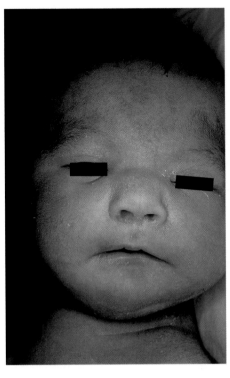

3.143

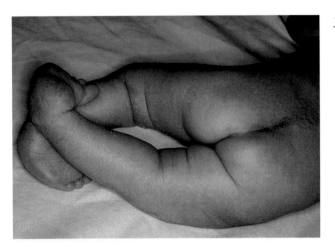

Figure 3.143. This infant has congenital dislocation of the right hip and the bilateral clubfoot. Note the asymmetric buttock creases typical of congenital dislocation of the hip. In Möbius' syndrome there may be deformities of the hands and feet and arthrogryposis is not uncommon.

Figure 3.142. A close-up of the face of the same infant. Note the mask-like facies, eyelid ptosis, and drooping of the angles of the mouth. These infants have inefficient sucking and swallowing. In Möbius' syndrome there are usually bilateral cranial nerve palsies involving the sixth and seventh cranial nerves. Occasionally other cranial nerves (three, five, nine and twelve) may be involved.

3.144

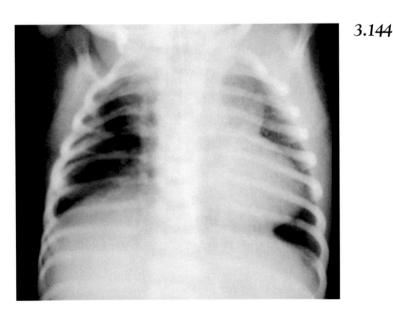

Figure 3.144. A chest radiograph in Poland's anomaly demonstrates the increased lucency of the right upper chest, especially of soft tissue, due to the absence of the pectoralis muscle. Compare the appearance of the scapulae on both sides. Note that the ribs are normal.

3.145

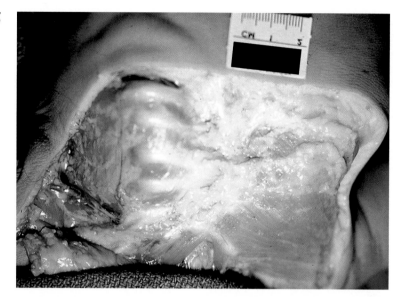

Figure 3.145. The pathologic appearance of the chest in an infant who had congenital absence of the pectoralis muscle.

3.146

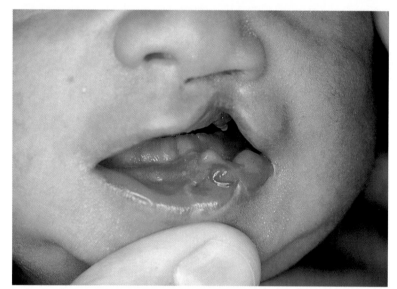

Figure 3.146. This infant with the popliteal pterygium syndrome (popliteal web syndrome) shows the unilateral cleft lip and cleft palate. There are lip pits and also note the remnants of the oral frenula which have been cut. Oral frenula are typically seen in these infants and there may be cutaneous webs between the eyelids.

3.147

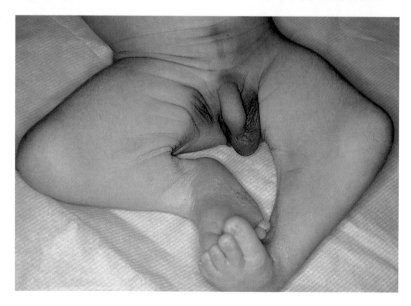

Figure 3.147. In the same infant note the very marked popliteal webbing which extends from the leg up to the thigh. Also note the divided scrotum with cryptorchidism on the right.

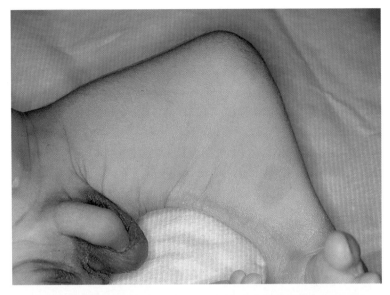

3.148

Figure 3.148. A close-up of the large popliteal web. The dense fibrous cord in the posterior portion of the popliteal pterygium may contain the tibial nerve.

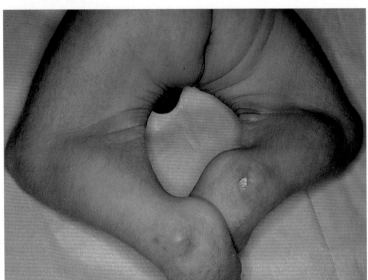

3.149

Figure 3.149. A posterior view of the lower extremities of the same infant shows the large popliteal pterygia extending from the hips to the ankles. There is also clubbing of both feet, a common finding in this condition.

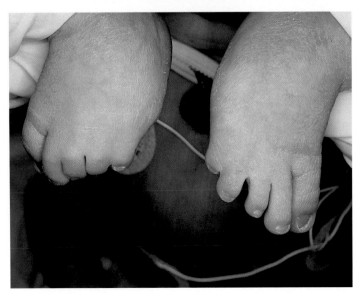

3.150

Figure 3.150. In the same infant there is syndactyly of the toes in both feet. Note the pyramidal form of the skin over the hallux which is typically seen in this condition.

3.151

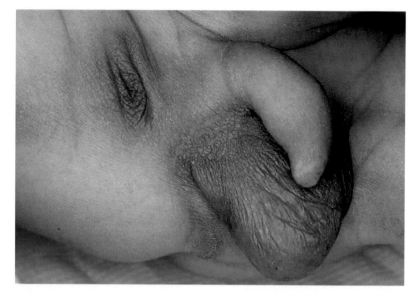

Figure 3.151. A close-up of the genitalia of the same infant as shown in Figure 3.150 shows the divided scrotum with cryptorchidism on the right. In female infants there may be hypoplastic labia minora and the genitalia may be ambiguous.

3.152

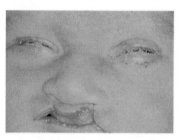 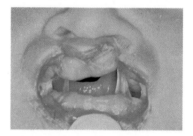

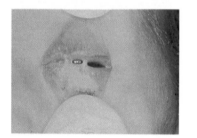 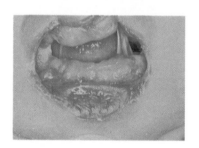

Figure 3.152. This female infant with popliteal pterygium syndrome presented with the filiform adhesions between the eyelids which are seen in 20% of patients. Cleft lip and palate are seen in 85% and pits of the lower lip are seen in 60%. The bands of tissue extending between the jaws which are well demonstrated in this patient are noted in about 35%.

3.153

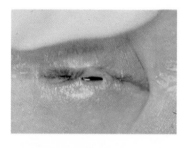 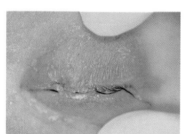

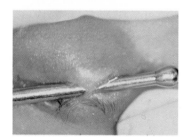 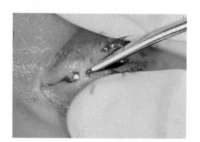

Figure 3.153. Close-up of the filiform adhesions between the eyelids of the same infant.

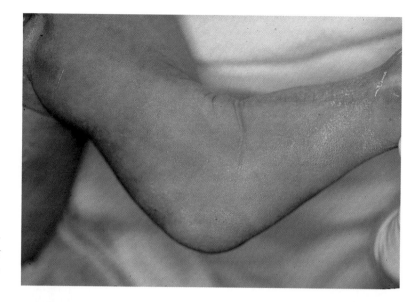

Figure 3.154. The popliteal ptery-gium in the same infant is not nearly as severe as in the previous example. Note the abnormal digits.

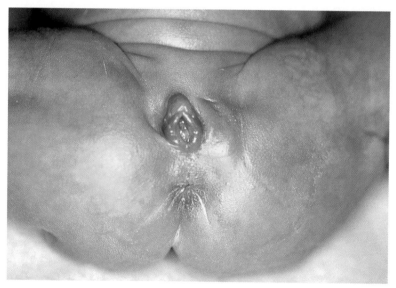

Figure 3.155. Absence of the labia majora is present in about 60% of infants with popliteal pterygium syndrome.

Figure 3.156. Prader-Willi syn-drome presents in the neonate with marked hypotonia, a weak cry, and hypogonadism at birth. In Prader-Willi syndrome the mother may note decreased fetal activity, and there is a breech presentation in about 30% of cases. Although born at term, the infants are usually small, weighing less than 3000 g. There is a charac-teristic history of feeding difficulty which may result in failure to thrive. The condition is sporadic and there is a preponderance of males. In Prader-Willi syndrome, the kary-otype is abnormal in about 50% of cases (deletion 15q).

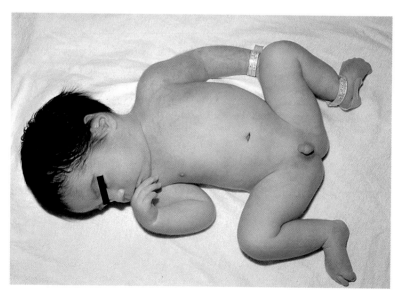

3.157

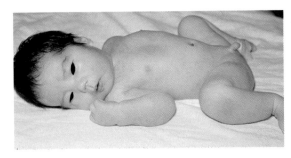

Figure 3.157. In this view of the same infant as in Figure 3.156, in addition to the hypotonia, some of the characteristic craniofacial features are apparent. Note the almond-shaped, upslanting palpebral fissures and the prominent forehead.

3.158

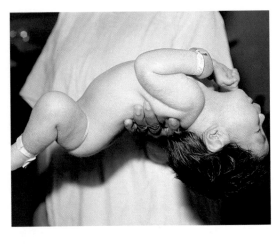

Figure 3.158. There is marked hypotonia in this infant with Prader-Willi syndrome in the prone position. It is usually severe in early infancy, and Moro's reflex and tendon reflexes are decreased or absent. Congenital dislocation of the hips is not uncommon.

3.159

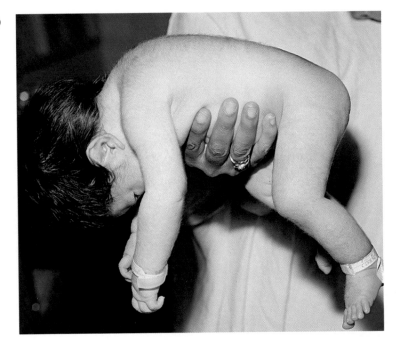

Figure 3.159. Marked hypotonia in this infant with Prader-Willi syndrome when the infant is held in the supine position.

3.160

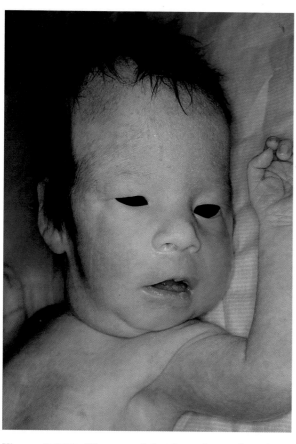

3.161

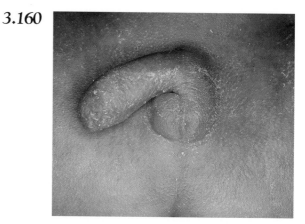

Figure 3.161. In the same infant note the cryptorchidism and a rudimentary scrotum.

Figure 3.160. Close-up of the face of an infant showing the characteristic craniofacial features. Note the prominent forehead and a reduced biparietal diameter. The eyes are almond shaped with upslanting palpebral fissures. The ears are dysplastic and the mouth is fish-like with a triangular upper lip. Note the small hand. The hands and feet may be small and remain small. Clinodactyly and syndactyly may be present in Prader-Willi syndrome.

Figure 3.162. In this term infant with progeria (Hutchinson-Gilford syndrome) there was marked growth retardation (birthweight 1800 g). The face is small with a large head (pseudohydrocephalus) and there is a marked lack of subcutaneous tissue and prominence of the knees. This is a condition in which there is pseudosenility with hypertension, cardiomegaly, and atherosclerosis resulting in early death (at the average age of 14 years).

3.162

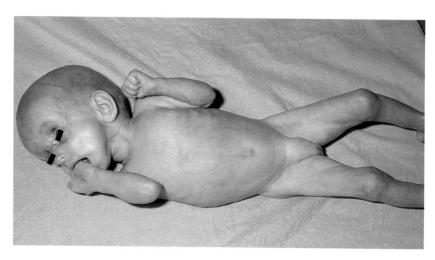

3.163

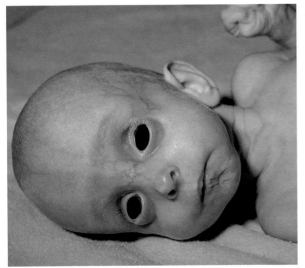

3.164

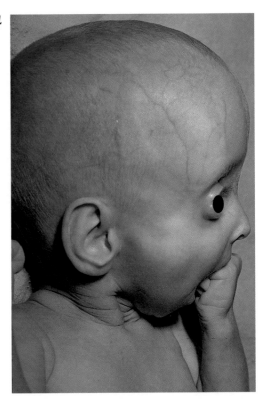

Figure 3.163. A close-up of the face of the same infant as shown in Figure 3.16 at age 6 weeks shows the small face with large head (pseudohydrocephalus), frontal and parietal bossing, hypotrichosis (scalp, eyebrows, and eyelashes), thin skin, prominent scalp veins, prominent eyes, mid-face hypoplasia, and micrognathia. The nose is thin and rather beaked.

Figure 3.164. Lateral view of the head and face in the same infant. Note the pseudohydrocephalus, hypotrichosis, prominent scalp veins, prominent eyes, small beak-like nose, and micrognathia. Note the prominent buccal pads in the cheek. These infants feed well and growth is normal until about the first year of life when it plateaus.

3.165

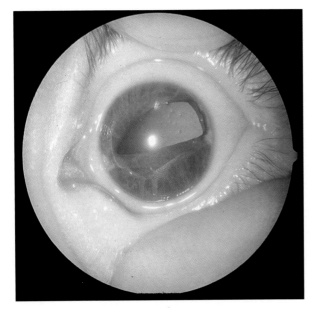

Figure 3.165. Rieger's syndrome is an autosomal dominant neural crest disorder in which there are abnormalities of the pituitary gland, teeth, and the mesenchymal structures of the eye. In this infant with Rieger's syndrome note the changes in the left eye. The pupil is distorted by peripheral anterior synechiae (adhesion of the iris to the cornea).

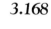

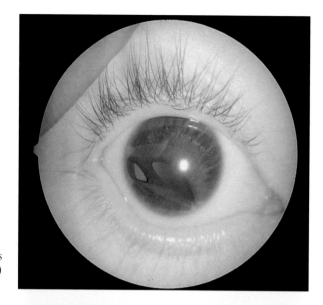

Figure 3.166. The same infant showing the changes in the right eye. Note the polycoria (multiple pupils) and peripheral anterior synechiae.

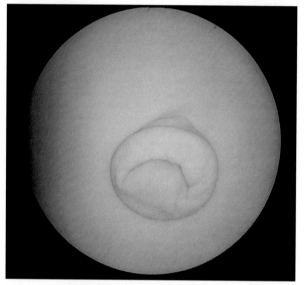

Figure 3.167. Patients with Rieger's syndrome have an unusually short umbilical cord which leaves a very characteristic umbilicus as seen in the same affected infant.

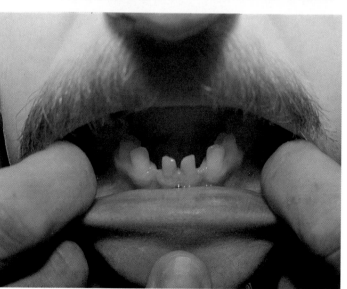

Figure 3.168. The father of the same infant shows hypodontia of the teeth. He also had ophthalmologic changes.

3.169

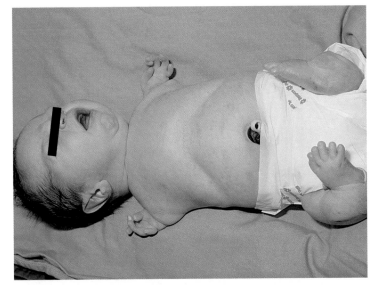

Figure 3.169. This infant with (pseudothalidomide syndrome) shows the tetraphocomelia. There is no cleft lip or palate, which would make the diagnosis the pseudothalidomide syndrome rather than Roberts' syndrome. The limb malformations are symmetric and more severe in the upper than in the lower limbs. Compare this infant to an infant exposed to maternal thalidomide in Volume I, Figure 3.23.

3.170

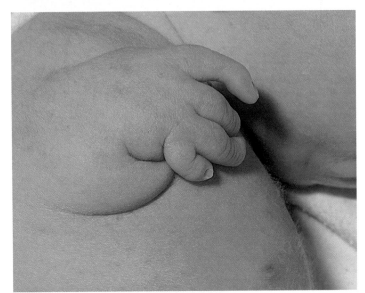

Figure 3.170. This is a close-up view of the right upper extremity of the infant. The phocomelia has resulted in absence of humeri, radii, and ulnae. In Roberts' syndrome the malformed hands may have hypoplastic or absent thumbs and there may be abnormalities of the digits.

3.171

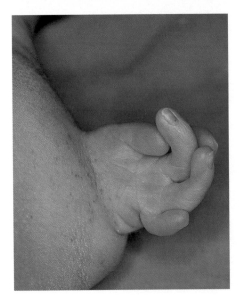

Figure 3.171. The left hand of the same infant showing the phocomelia with the abnormal hand and digits.

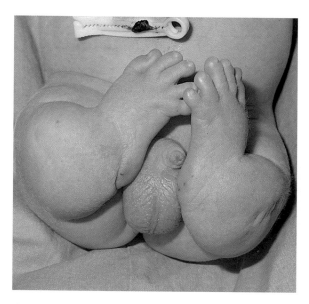

3.172

Figure 3.172. The lower extremities of the infant show the less severe changes in that the femora, tibiae, and fibulae are hypoplastic and the feet are abnormal.

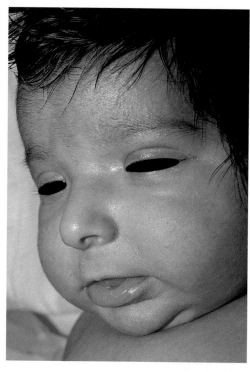

3.173

Figure 3.173. This infant with Rubenstein-Taybi syndrome presented at term with a birthweight of 2700 g and a length of 48 cm. Note the prominent forehead, hypertrichosis, downslanting palpebral fissures, epicanthic folds, long eyelashes, hypertelorism, broad nasal bridge, a beaked nose with a nasal septum extending below the alae nasi, and micrognathia. In addition to the findings above, patients with Rubenstein-Taybi syndrome commonly have microcephaly, low-set malformed ears and a high arched narrow palate.

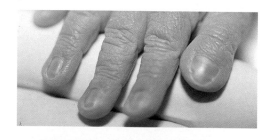

3.174

Figure 3.174. This figure shows the typical broad thumbs and broad toes which are seen in all infants with Rubenstein-Taybi syndrome. There may be shortening of thumbs and big toes. Clinodactyly of the fifth finger and overlapping of toes are seen in about 50% of these infants.

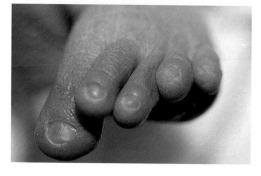

3.175

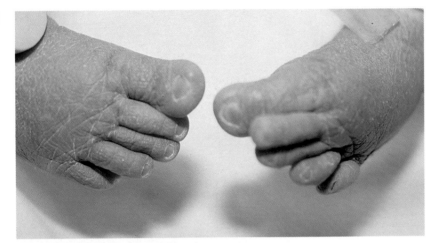

Figure 3.175. Broad thumbs and broad toes in another infant with Rubenstein-Taybi syndrome. Note the typical overlapping of toes.

3.176

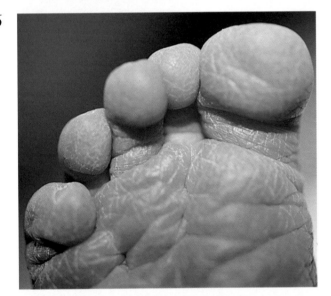

Figure 3.176. Another view of the same infant with the Rubenstein-Taybi syndrome showing the large big toe and overlapping of toes.

3.177

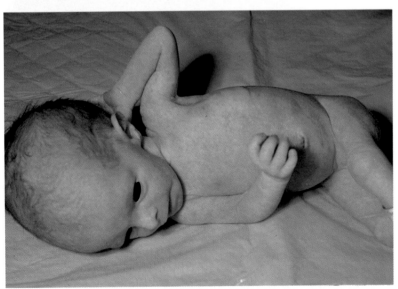

Figure 3.177. This term baby shows the typical findings of Russell-Silver syndrome in that he was unusually small for his gestational age (less than the 3rd percentile), small in stature, and had pseudohydrocephalus in that the head appeared to be disproportionately large for the small face. The proximal extremities are relatively short and the distal extremities are long (disproportionate dwarfism). Some of these infants may have skeletal asymmetry which may involve the entire body (hemihypertrophy) or which may be limited to involve only the skull or a limb.

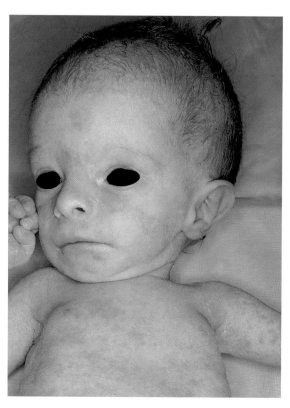

3.178

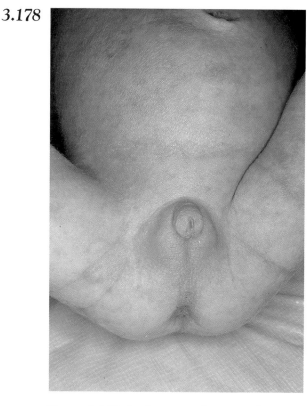

3.179

Figure 3.178. Close-up of the face of the same infant showing again the disproportion between the large head and the small face which tapers to a narrow jaw giving rise to a triangular facies. The fronto-occipital circumference is normal and the fontanelles are enlarged. Note the frontal bossing, prominent eyes, long eyelashes, and downturned angles of the mouth (giving a carp-like appearance), micrognathia, and posteriorly rotated ears.

A triangular facies is often the result of a disparity between the growth of the cranium, paced by normal brain growth, and the growth of the facial skeleton whose bones may share in an intrinsic growth deficiency.

Figure 3.179. In the same infant note the cryptorchidism. Genital hypoplasia and hypogonadism are commonly present in Russell-Silver syndrome.

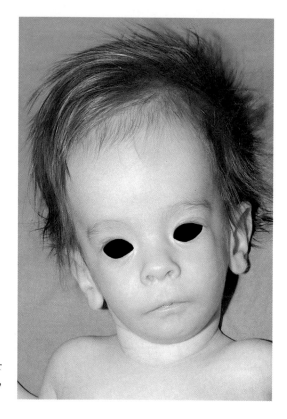

3.180

Figure 3.180. In another infant with the Russell-Silver syndrome, note the pseudohydrocephalus, prominent eyes, triangular facies, and carp-like mouth.

3.181

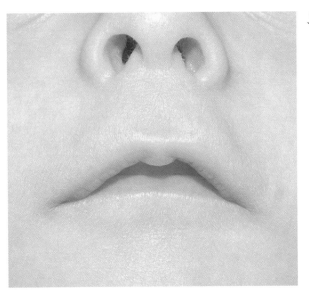

Figure 3.181. Close-up view of the mouth of the same infant as in Figure 3.180 showing the typical carp-like or inverted V-shaped appearance of the mouth.

3.182

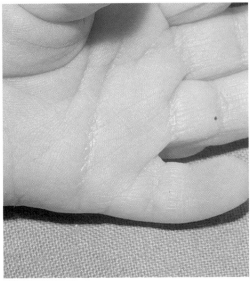

Figure 3.182. The same infant had a single palmar crease and clinodactyly of the fifth finger, which are also common findings in Russell-Silver syndrome.

3.183

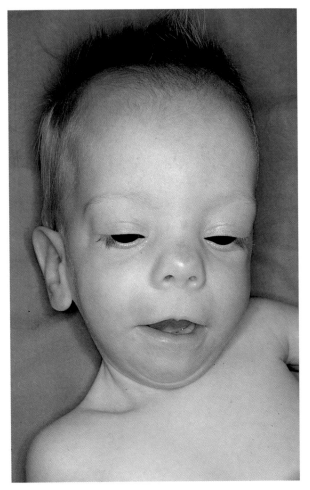

Figure 3.183. In the Smith-Lemli-Opitz syndrome the infants are small for their gestational age with a mean birthweight of 2560 g at term, commonly present as breech presentations, and have mental retardation. This is a female infant, but male infants predominate. There is microcephaly with moderate scaphocephaly, bilateral ptosis, low-set ears, a broad nasal tip with anteverted nostrils, and mild micrognathia. Other findings that may occur are an antimongoloid slant and epicanthic folds of the eyes.

3.184

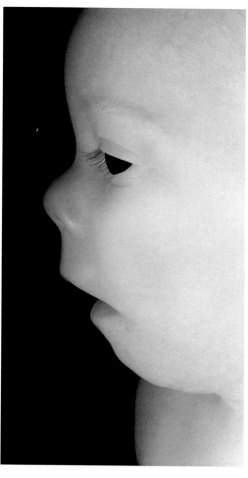

3.185

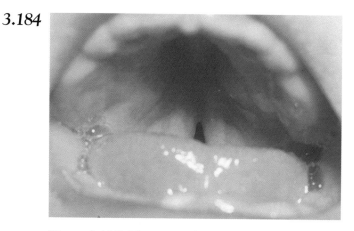

Figure 3.185. The same infant with Smith-Lemli-Opitz syndrome had a small cleft in the soft palate.

Figure 3.184. Lateral view of the face of the same infant. Note the long eyelashes, the ptosis of the eyelids, anteverted nostrils and the mild micrognathia.

3.186

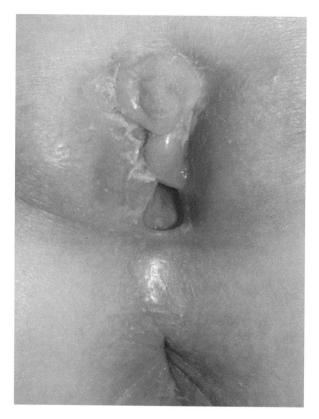

Figure 3.186. Note the hypoplastic genitalia. Males have small penises and hypogonadism.

3.187

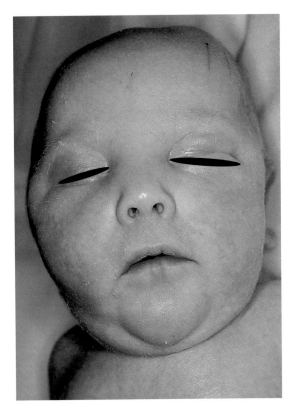

3.188

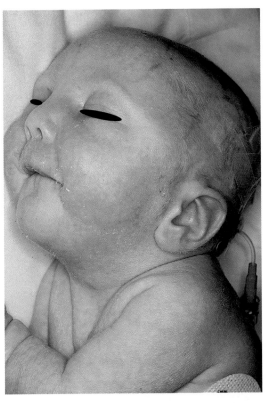

Figure 3.187. Another example of Smith-Lemli-Opitz syndrome in a male infant showing the typical appearance of the face. Note the microcephaly, closed eyes associated with ptosis, inner epicanthic folds, broad nasal tip with anteverted nostrils, and micrognathia.

Figure 3.188. The same infant from the lateral view showing the face and head. Note the microcephaly with a tendency to scaphocephaly, low-set ears, ptosis, anteverted nostrils, and micrognathia.

3.189

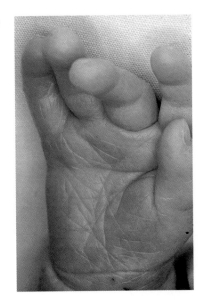 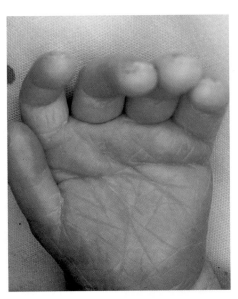

Figure 3.189. The hands of the same infant. The figure on the left shows a single palmar crease on the right hand and the figure on the right shows a Sydney line on the left hand. A Sydney line is often reported as a single palmar crease but note that there are two separate transverse palmar creases which are joined by another crease. These palmar findings are common in many normal infants and are seen in many syndromes.

3.190

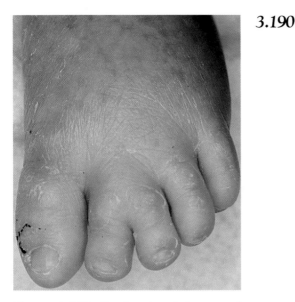

Figure 3.190. Syndactyly of the second and third toes is a common finding in Smith-Lemli-Opitz syndrome, but may occur in normal patients or in many other syndromes.

3.191

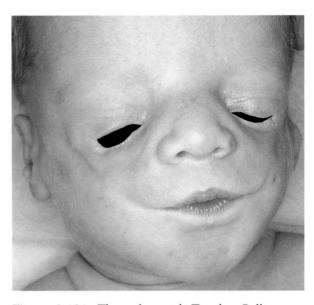

Figure 3.191. This infant with Treacher-Collins syndrome (mandibulofacial dysostosis) shows the typical findings of antimongoloid slanting palpebral fissures, colobomas of the lateral part of the lower eyelids, deficient eyelashes, hypoplasia of the zygomatic arch, micrognathia, and malformed ears. The nose is prominent.

3.192

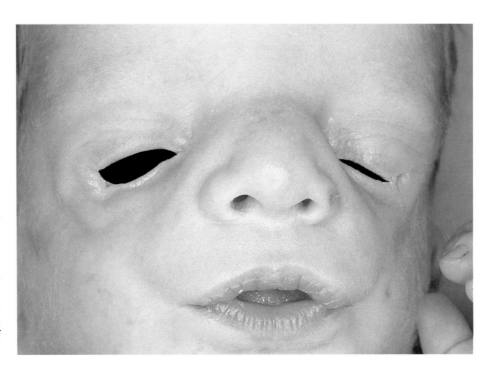

Figure 3.192. Close-up of the face of the same infant showing the antimongoloid slant and colobomas of the lower eyelids which typically occur at the junction of the inner two-thirds and outer third of the lower eyelids. Note the absence of eyebrows and eyelashes, the prominent nose and the hypoplasia of the zygomatic bone.

3.193

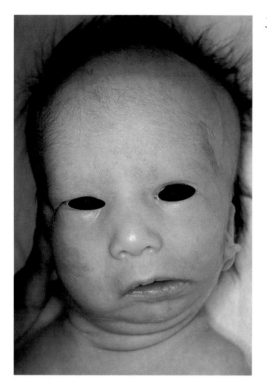

3.194

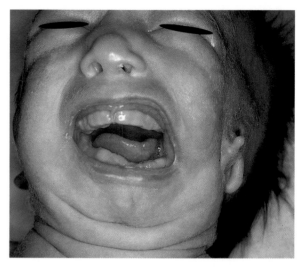

Figure 3.194. The same infant when crying better demonstrates the findings. Note the antimongoloid slant, the prominent nose, and the micrognathia. Infants with this syndrome may have a cleft of the palate, particularly of the soft palate. A finding in many of these infants is a projection of the scalp hair onto the lateral cheek.

Figure 3.193. A less severe case of Treacher-Collins syndrome. Note the unilateral macrostomia and the abnormal ear. Treacher-Collins syndrome is a familial malformation involving structures originating from the first branchial arch and may have moderate expressivity.

3.195

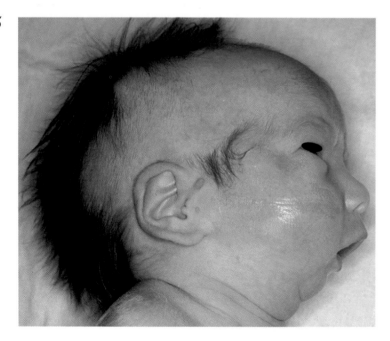

Figure 3.195. A lateral view of the same infant showing the slightly abnormal right ear with preauricular skin tags, the prominent nose and micrognathia.

3.196

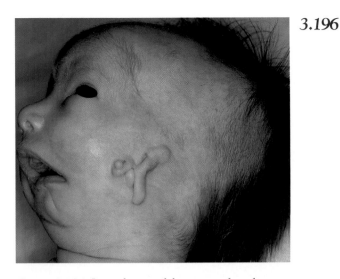

3.197

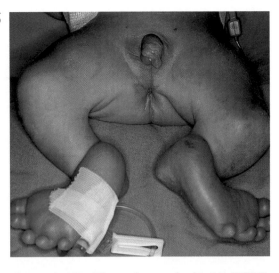

Figure 3.196. Lateral view of the same infant showing the grossly abnormal ear on the left side with atresia of the auditory canal, the antimongoloid slant, prominent nose and micrognathia.

Figure 3.197. This infant with the VACTERL syndrome exhibits the following: *v*ertebral anomalies, imperforate *a*nus, *c*ardiac defects, *t*racheo*e*sophageal fistula, *r*enal anomalies, and *l*imb defects. In cases where the acronym VATER is used, the "C" for cardiac abnormalities, and the "L" for limb defects are excluded, and the "R" stands for renal and radial anomalies. This infant had a tracheoesophageal fistula, duodenal atresia, and anal stenosis. There was a double outlet left ventricle causing congestive failure, hydronephrosis, ambiguous genitalia, and cryptorchidism. There was sacral dysgenesis and hemivertebrae, absence of the radii bilaterally, absence of tibiae bilaterally, and severe clubfoot.

3.198

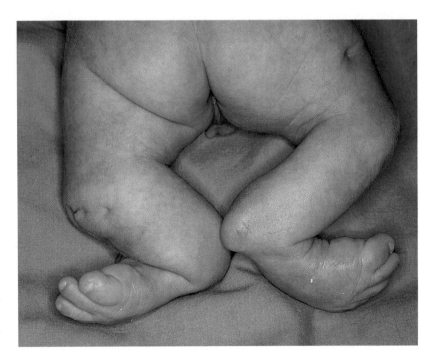

Figure 3.198. A posterior view of the pelvis and lower extremities of the same infant. Note the abnormal gluteal folds, as this infant also had bilateral dislocation of the hips. Note the skin dimples at the joints.

3.199

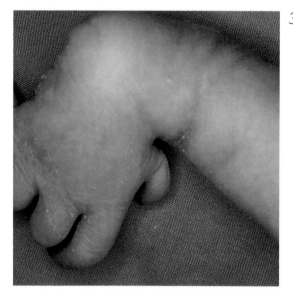

Figure 3.199. The right upper extremity of this same infant shown in Figures 3.197 and 3.198 shows the club hand due to the absence of the radius.

3.200

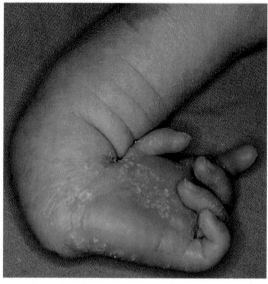

Figure 3.200. The left upper extremity of the same infant shows the absence of the radius, resulting in a club hand. Also note the abnormal thumb.

3.201

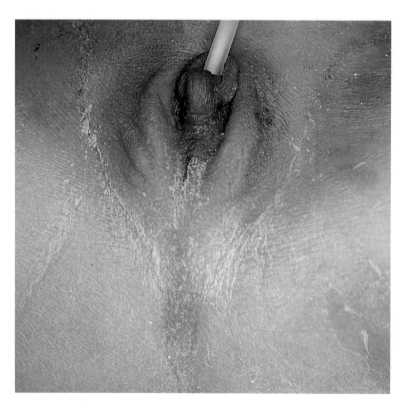

Figure 3.201. This infant with the VACTERL syndrome presented with vertebral anomalies of the lower thoracic vertebrae, an esophageal atresia, dextrocardia, imperforate anus, and ambiguous genitalia. There were no anomalies of the limbs. Note the imperforate anus and ambiguous genitalia. Karyotype was normal XX. A catheter placed in the single perineal opening appeared in the colostomy. This confirmed the presence of a cloacal sac.

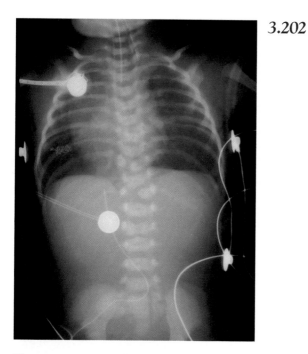

3.202

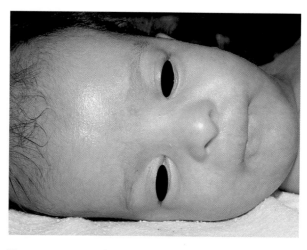

3.203

Figure 3.202. Radiograph of this infant shows the air-filled blind esophageal sac. Note that there is no communicating fistula, as the abdomen is completely opaque due to lack of air in the GI tract. There is abnormal segmentation of the distal thoracic vertebrae and anomalies of the ribs.

Figure 3.203. Infants with Zellweger syndrome (cerebrohepatorenal syndrome) present with hypotonia and typical craniofacial features, in addition to other finings. In the close-up of the head of this infant note the high prominent forehead and somewhat flattened facies, hypertelorism, epicanthic folds, anteverted nares, and micrognathia.

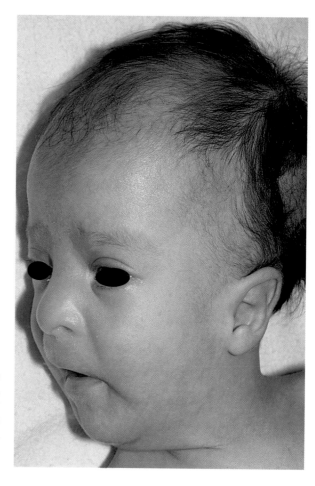

3.204

Figure 3.204. The lateral view of the face of the same infant shows the high forehead, flattened facies, micrognathia, and low-set ears. There is brachycephaly as the occiput is flat. In this infant the fontanelles were wide open, and hepatosplenomegaly, albuminuria, and ulnar deviation with a simian crease of the hand were present.

3.205

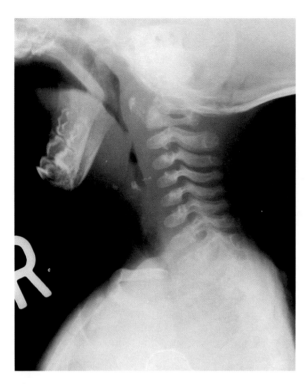

Figure 3.205. Stippling of the epiphyses and hyoid are common in Zellweger syndrome. This radiograph of the neck shows stippling at the hyoid bone.

3.206

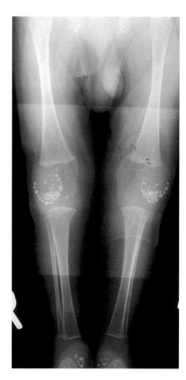

Figure 3.206. Early punctate mineralization of the patella is a common finding, and note the stippling at the knee joints and ankles.

3.207

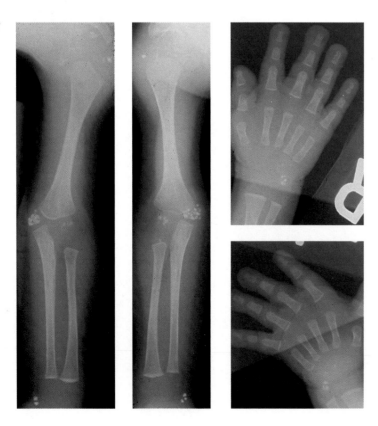

Figure 3.207. Radiographs of the upper extremities of the same infant showing the stippling at the elbows and wrists.

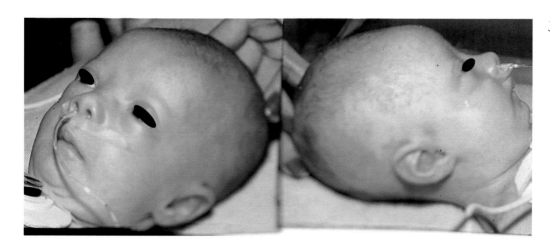

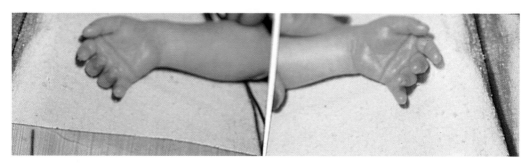

Figure 3.208. This infant with Zellweger syndrome had marked hypotonia and shows the typical appearance of the head and face, the single palmar creases, and clinodactyly. There is commonly ulnar deviation with simian creases of the hand. Brushfield's spots also occur in infants with Zellweger syndrome. Because of the hypotonia, craniofacial findings, Brushfield's spots, and simian creases, these infants often are mistaken for infants with trisomy 21.

Chapter 4
Chromosomal Disorders

Chromosomal abnormalities are fairly common. They occur in about 1 in every 200 deliveries, although many of these infants are phenotypically normal. In addition, 50% of all spontaneous abortions involve a chromosomal abnormality. Nondisjunction, where an extra chromosome (or part of a chromosome) is present (e.g., trisomy 21), is the most common cause of chromosomal disorders. Translocation syndromes, where chromosomal material breaks off from one chromosome and translocates to another, may not have classic clinical findings and may be difficult to diagnose. Usually infants with balanced translocations are only carriers and do not demonstrate clinical manifestations, while unbalanced translocations result in clinical signs. A deletion occurs when chromosomal material is missing from either the upper (p) or lower (q) arms of a chromosome (e.g., cri du chat syndrome with deletion of the upper short arm of chromosome 5 5p–). An abnormal number of X or Y chromosomes can also result in significant clinical syndromes (e.g., Turner's syndrome with absence of one of the X chromosomes 45X0). Chromosomal analysis should be considered for all stillbirths, newborns with multiple congenital anomalies, or to confirm a suspected chromosomal diagnosis.

4.1

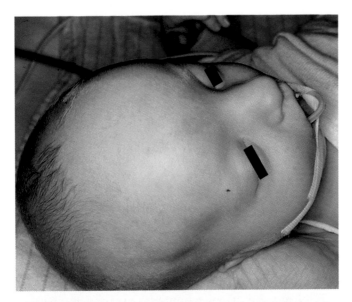

Figure 4.1. In the syndrome caused by deletion of the short arm of chromosome number 4 (4p– syndrome, Wolf-Hirschhorn syndrome), there is marked prenatal growth deficiency and decreased fetal activity. At birth the facial features are typical: microcephaly, a high forehead, prominent glabella, and a wide nasal bridge with nasal beaking (the "Grecian helmet" appearance of the head). This infant also has craniofacial asymmetry.

4.2

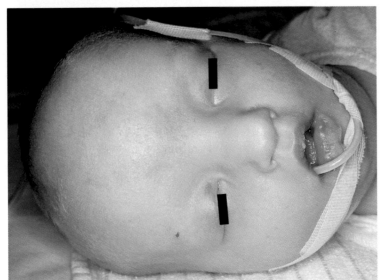

Figure 4.2. A frontal view of the same infant shows the high forehead and a prominent glabella. The eyebrows are highly arched and sparse medially. There is nasal beaking and epicanthic folds with bilateral ptosis. There is a short deep philtrum with a short upper lip and a turned-down, fish-like mouth. A cleft lip and/or palate occurs in about 10% of these infants.

4.3

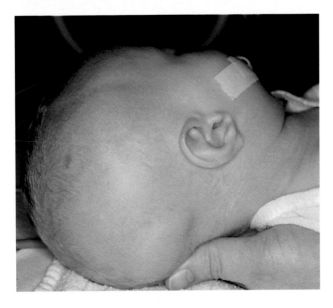

Figure 4.3. In the lateral view of the same infant note the lobeless pinnae and micrognathia. The external auditory canals are narrow.

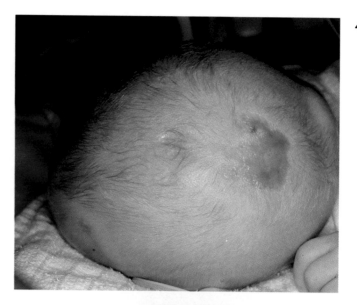

4.4

Figure 4.4. This same infant with Wolf-Hirschhorn syndrome had a posterior midline scalp defect which is seen in about 10% of these infants. He also had hypospadias and cryptorchidism, a finding frequently associated with this syndrome.

Other findings in infants with this syndrome include coloboma of the iris, simian crease, hypoplastic dermal ridges, talipes equinovarus, and cardiac anomalies. Radiologically there may be fusion of the ribs and dislocation of the hips.

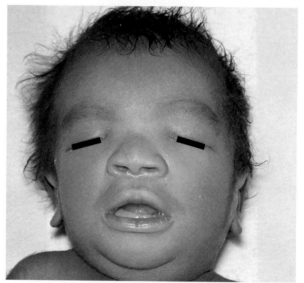

4.5

Figure 4.5. Deletion of the short arm of chromosome number 5 (5p– syndrome, cri du chat syndrome) is present in this infant; his twin was normal. Note the craniofacial disproportion, with microcephaly, round face, dysplastic low-set ears, the downward (antimongoloid) slant of the palpebral fissures, hypertelorism, and micrognathia. The typical cat cry (high-pitched mewing cry) was present. The cat cry is due to a narrow larynx, and occurs as a result of the cords being approximated anteriorly leaving a narrow opening posteriorly. It is not present in all infants and disappears as the infant grows.

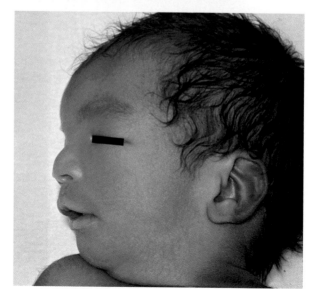

4.6

Figure 4.6. The lateral view of the same infant shows the low-set ears, flattened nose, and micrognathia.

4.7

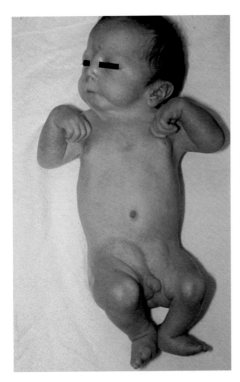

4.8

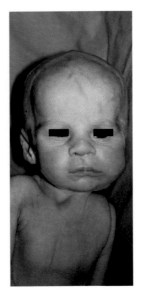 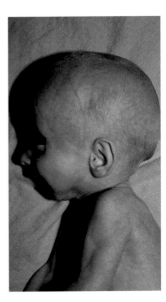

Figure 4.8. Another infant with trisomy 8 shows the dysplastic craniofacial features (short nose, broad nasal bridge, prominent nares, wide philtrum, thin upper lip, and low-set ears with thick helices).

Figure 4.7. Trisomy 8 syndrome is usually a trisomy 8/normal mosaicism. Note the dysmorphic craniofacial features, micrognathia, postural deformity of the hands, cryptorchidism with bilateral inguinal herniae, and absence of the patellae.

4.9

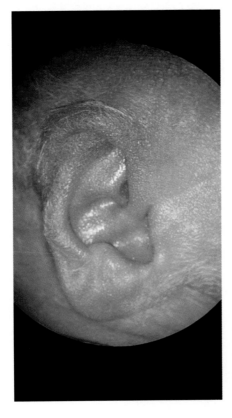 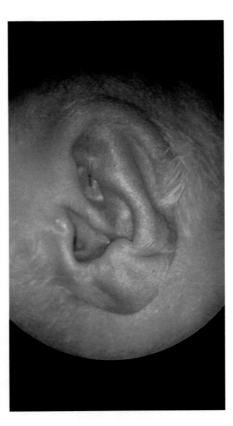

Figure 4.9. A close-up view of the ears of the same infant demonstrates the thick helices.

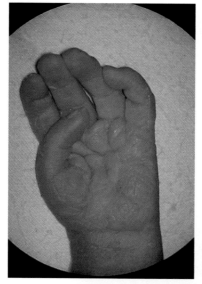
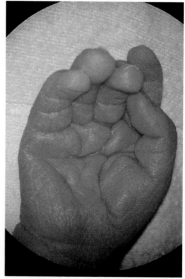

4.10

Figure 4.10. The hands of the same infant with trisomy 8 show the shortened hallux, camptodactyly, and deep flexion creases of the palms. Deep furrows are found on both the palms of the hand and soles of the feet (these regress with increasing age).

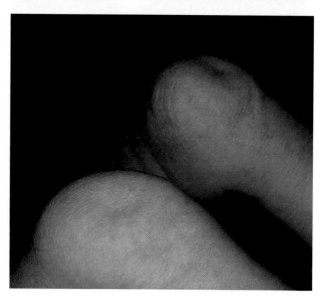

4.11

Figure 4.11. Congenital absence of the patellae is another finding in the trisomy 8 syndrome. In addition to the findings shown here in trisomy 8 other common findings include cleft palate, single palmar crease, and contractures of large joints.

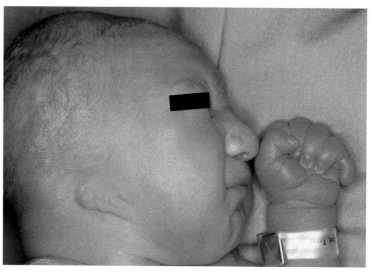

4.12

Figure 4.12. In the trisomy 13 syndrome (Patau's syndrome) there is microcephaly, a sloping forehead, grossly abnormal ears, micrognathia, and polydactyly. In this infant, in addition to these findings, there was a scalp defect and atresia of the external auditory canals. In trisomy 13 syndrome other findings include microphthalmia, anophthalmia, hypo- or hypertelorism, depressed nasal bridge, bilateral cleft lip and/or palate, congenital heart disease, omphalocele, large umbilical hernia, renal anomalies, flexion and overlapping of the fingers, single palmar crease, and a prominent heel giving rise to "rocker-bottom" feet. If the infant sur-

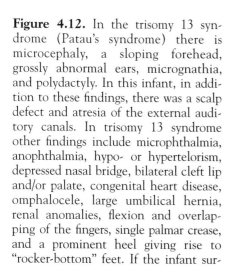

4.13

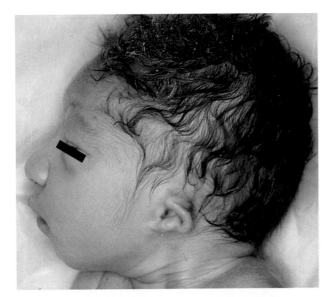

Figure 4.13. Trisomy 13 in another infant showing microcephaly, microtia with low-set ears, and micrognathia. This same infant had bilateral glaucoma.

4.14

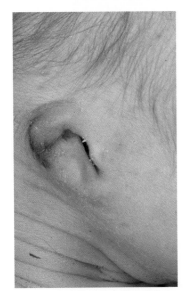
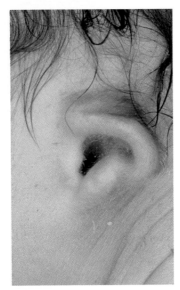

Figure 4.14. A close-up view of the ears of the same infant showing the bilateral microtia. Ear abnormalities may be minimal or there may be total absence of the external auditory canal.

4.15

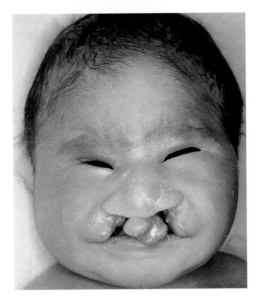

Figure 4.15. A common finding in trisomy 13 is bilateral cleft lip and palate. In this infant there is microcephaly, hypotelorism, the eyes are microphthalmic, and there is a receding forehead. On further study the infant had an alobar holoprosencephaly. In trisomy 13, central nervous system abnormalities are found in 50% or more of infants and, hence, one should check for a holoprosencephaly defect.

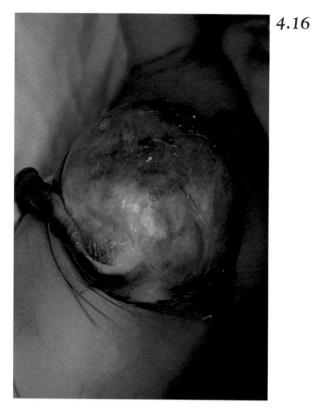

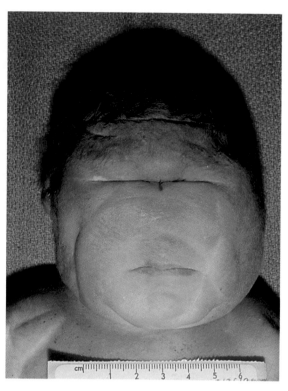

Figure 4.16. The same infant also had an omphalocele. The finding of cleft lip and palate with an omphalocele or large umbilical hernia should alert one to the possibility of the diagnosis of trisomy 13.

Figure 4.17. Median cleft syndrome may be associated with chromosomal defects. This infant with trisomy 13 had cyclops with anophthalmia. There is no proboscis present. There was arhinencephaly and alobar holoprosencephaly on CT scan.

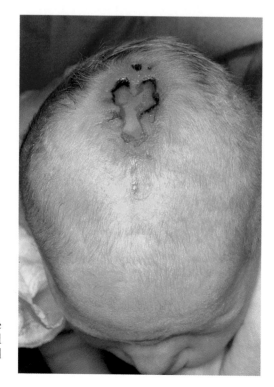

Figure 4.18. Another common finding in trisomy 13 is a midline scalp defect, which is most common in the parieto-occipital area. This infant also had abnormal ears, micrognathia, and polydactyly.

4.19

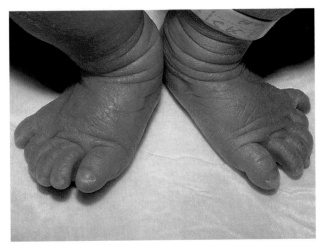

Figure 4.19. Polydactyly of the hands and feet occur frequently in infants with trisomy 13.

4.20

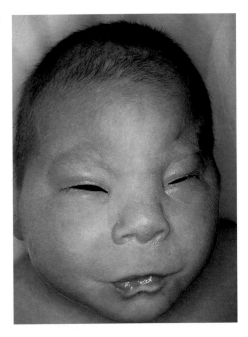

Figure 4.20. In this infant with trigonocephaly, hypotelorism, patchy alopecia, and eleven ribs, the diagnosis was that of a ring D chromosome defect (karyotype was performed in the pre-banding era). Trigonocephaly is associated with premature fusion of the metopic suture and may occur in chromosomal anomalies and in median cleft syndrome, but also occurs in normal infants.

4.21

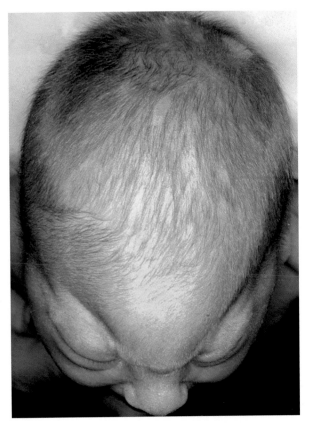

Figure 4.21. This view better demonstrates the trigonocephaly and the patchy alopecia.

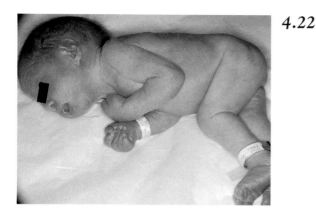

4.22

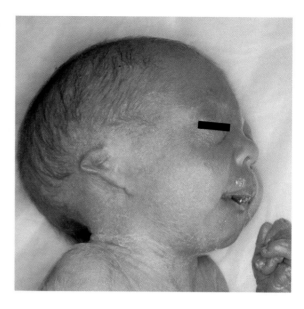

4.23

Figure 4.22. Severe intrauterine growth retardation (birthweight 1590 g at term) was noted in this infant with the typical findings of trisomy 18 (Edwards' syndrome). Note the low-set, poorly developed ears, micrognathia, and the typical overlapping position of the fingers. In trisomy 18 there is a preponderance of three females to one male infant. Other findings in trisomy 18 include prominent occiput, microcephaly, short sternum, congenital heart disease, abnormal genitalia, and renal anomalies (horseshoe kidney, polycystic kidneys, etc.). If the infant survives, there is severe mental retardation.

Figure 4.23. A close-up view of the face and skull in the same infant shows the characteristic prominent occiput, low-set abnormal ears with atresia of the external auditory canals (the ears often appear cupped), and micrognathia. The typical flexion deformity of the fingers can also be seen.

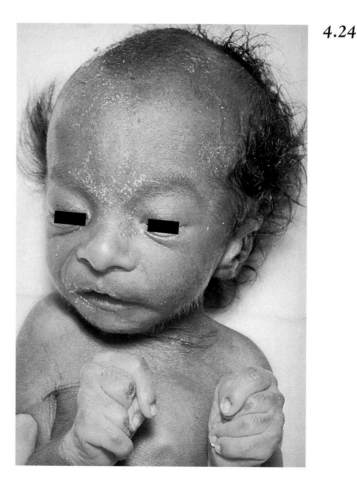

4.24

Figure 4.24. Trisomy 18 in another infant shows the intrauterine growth retardation, narrow bifrontal diameter, low-set ears, and micrognathia. Note the typical clenched hands with flexion deformities of the fingers.

4.25

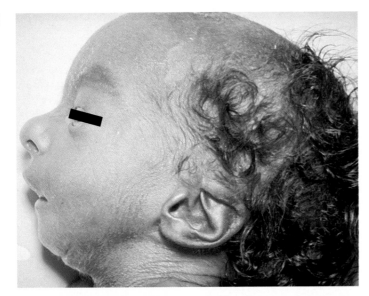

Figure 4.25. The lateral view of the same infant as in Fig. 4.24 shows the prominent occiput, low-set ears with a large pinna, and micrognathia.

4.26

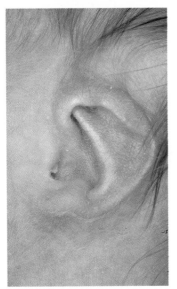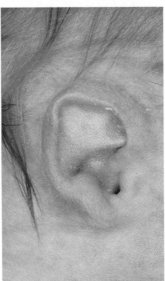

Figure 4.26. The right ear in this infant demonstrates the characteristic cupping ("tulip-shaped") deformity noted in infants with trisomy 18.

4.27

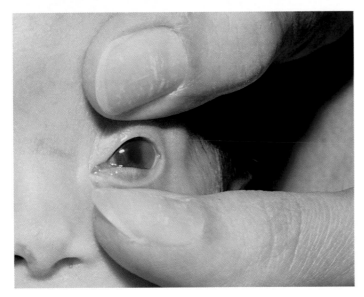

Figure 4.27. Coloboma of the left eye of this infant with trisomy 18. Other ophthalmologic findings in trisomy 18 include short palpebral fissures, hypoplasia of the orbital ridges, and corneal opacities.

4.28

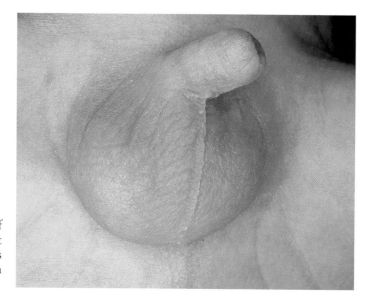

Figure 4.28. In trisomy 18, abnormalities of the genitalia are common. This male infant has cryptorchidism, and in female infants there may be hypoplasia of the labia majora with a prominent clitoris.

4.29

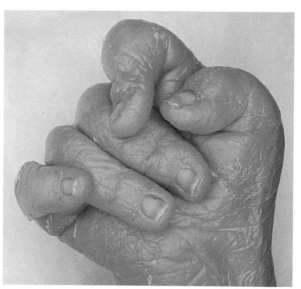

Figure 4.29. The appearance of this hand is very typical of infants with trisomy 18, occurring in about 50% of affected infants. Note the clenched hand with a tendency for the index finger to overlap the third and for the fifth finger to overlap the fourth. At times these fingers are extended, giving the appearance of the sign for "I love you" in American sign language. Infants with trisomy 18 also commonly have hypoplasia of the nails on both the fingers (especially the fifth finger) and the toes.

4.30

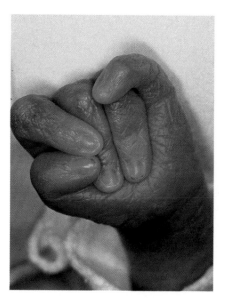
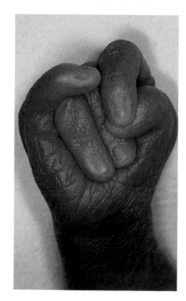

Figure 4.30. Another typical example of the hands in an infant with trisomy 18.

4.31

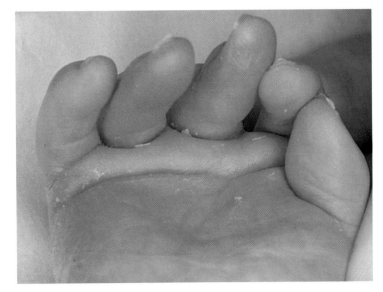

Figure 4.31. Note the single palmar crease in this infant with trisomy 18. A single palmar crease is a common finding in normal infants and is also noted in numerous syndromes. Note the lack of development of other dermal creases, indicating that there was a lack of fetal movement from early in gestation. In this infant there is an absence of finger creases on all fingers. In trisomy 18 it is not uncommon to have an absence of distal creases on the fifth finger (clinodactyly) and less commonly on the fourth and third fingers.

4.32

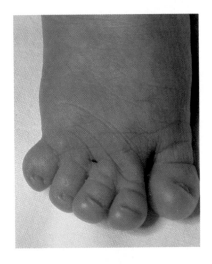 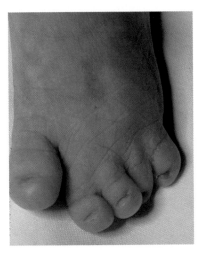

Figure 4.32. Note the short big toes and hypoplastic nails which are typically seen in trisomy 18. The short big toes are frequently dorsiflexed. There is also syndactyly of the second and third toes bilaterally in this infant, which is a common finding in normal infants and in infants with other pathologies, and is also reported in trisomy 18. Infants with trisomy 18 may have talipes equinovarus or "rocker-bottom" feet.

4.33

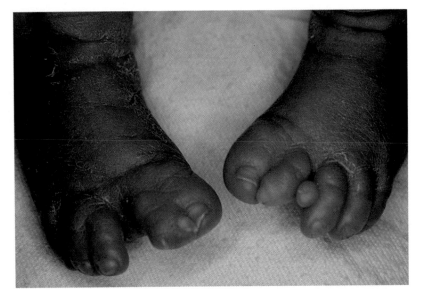

Figure 4.33. This infant did not have the typical clinical appearance of an infant with trisomy 18, but the radiographic findings of gracile ribs and antimongoloid pelvis were diagnostic. The diagnosis was confirmed by karyotype. Note the central polydactyly of the left foot and syndactyly of the right foot. Central polydactyly is an uncommon finding in normal infants and should alert one to the possible diagnosis of a chromosomal disorder.

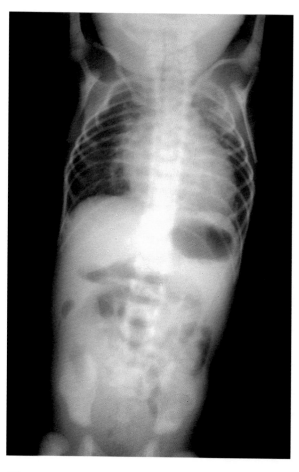

4.34

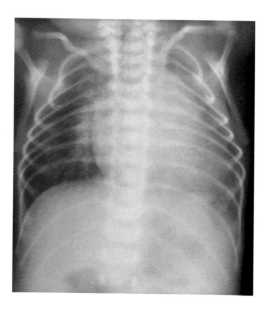

4.35

Figure 4.35. The chest radiograph of the same infant shows the gracile appearance of the ribs and the long slender clavicles, giving rise to the so-called "bicycle handle" clavicles. This radiologic appearance should always alert one to the possible diagnosis of trisomy 18.

Figure 4.34. This full-body radiograph illustrates the typical findings in trisomy 18. Note the gracile (fine, delicate) ribs and the antimongoloid (very vertical) appearance of the pelvis. The infant also had cardiac enlargement which was associated with congenital heart disease (patent ductus arteriosus).

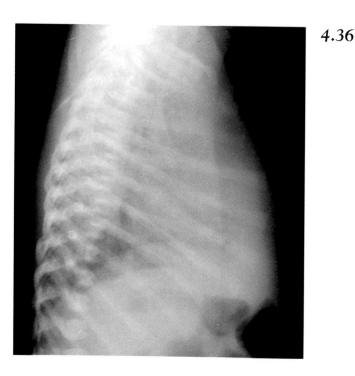

4.36

Figure 4.36. The sternum is short in trisomy 18, and sternal ossification centers are absent or decreased in number. In this lateral radiograph of the chest in another infant with trisomy 18, there are no sternal ossification centers.

4.37

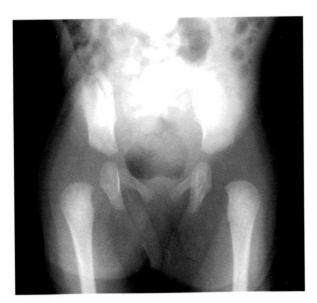

Figure 4.37. Radiograph of the pelvis in the same infant as shown in Figure 4.36 with trisomy 18 demonstrates the antimongoloid configuration. The pelvis is small, the iliac crest is narrow, and there are large acetabular angles.

4.38

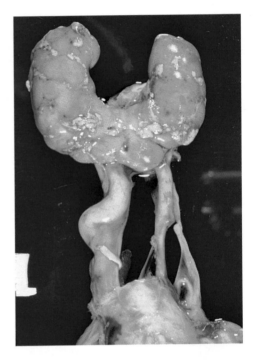

Figure 4.38. A pathologic specimen of a horseshoe kidney from an infant with trisomy 18. Note the hydroureter and hydronephrosis on the left. Horseshoe kidneys, ectopic kidneys, double ureters, and other renal anomalies are common in trisomy 18.

4.39

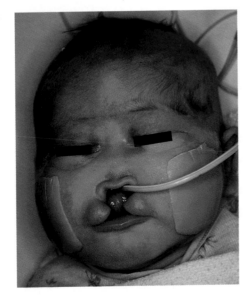

Figure 4.39. This infant with a median cleft, hypotelorism, and holoprosencephaly had an 18p– chromosomal defect. The most consistent features of the 18p– defect are ptosis, epicanthal folds, hypotelorism, rounded facies, and large protruding ears. In some cases, holoprosencephaly may be present. The hands and feet are relatively small. If the infant survives, there is severe mental retardation.

4.40

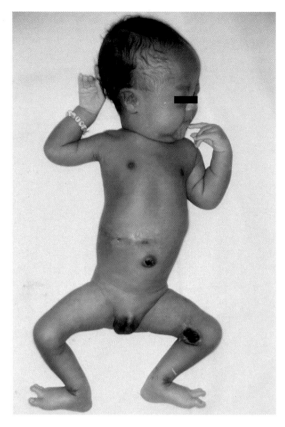

Figure 4.40. The typical appearance of an infant with trisomy 21 (Down syndrome). Note the marked hypotonia, flat facies, single palmar crease and separation of the first and second toes. The abdominal surgery was for the common finding of duodenal atresia. There is a burn at the left knee which occurred during surgery. The incidence of trisomy 21 is 1 in 700 newborns. The typical findings in trisomy 21 include hypotonia, poor Moro's reflex, hyperflexibility of joints, excess skin at the back of the neck, a flat facial profile, slanted palpebral fissures, dysplasia of the pelvis, and hand and feet abnormalities.

4.41

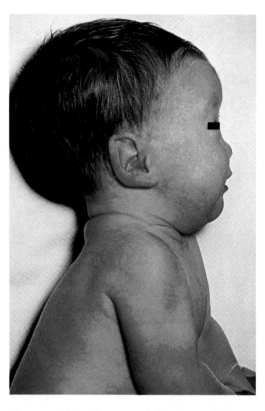

Figure 4.41. The typical flat facies ("glatte-gesicht") in an infant with trisomy 21 is due to a lack of the orbital ridges, a flat nose, and micrognathia, which together result in a lack of profile. Also note that there is some excess skin at the nape of the neck.

4.42

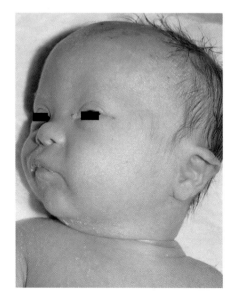

Figure 4.42. In trisomy 21 the head is small and round (brachycephaly) which occurs as a result of the flat occiput and the flat facies (compare with the prominent occiput seen in trisomy 18 [Figure 4.25]). There is a mongoloid appearance to the eyes due to the slanting palpebral fissures, the ears are low set, the nose is flat, and there is micrognathia.

4.43

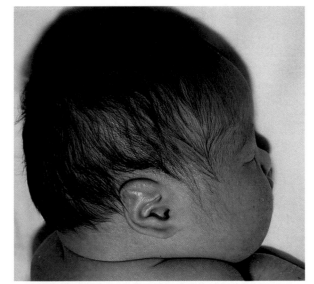

Figure 4.43. Trisomy 21 in another infant showing the typical flat facial features, flat occiput, and webbing of the neck. There was also mild microcephaly.

4.44

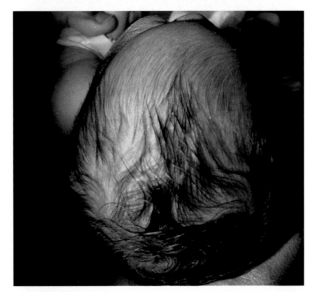

Figure 4.44. A view of the same infant's head shows the brachycephaly which results from the flat forehead and flat occiput. The sutures were normal.

4.45

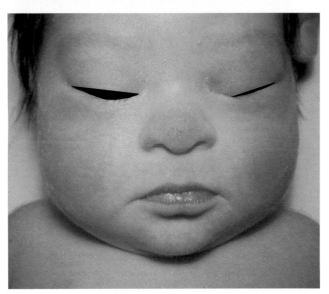

Figure 4.45. A close-up of the face of an infant with trisomy 21 shows the characteristic mongolian slant of the eyes, the hypertelorism, and the flat nose. Epicanthal folds, a common finding in Down syndrome, may be less obvious in the neonate than later in life. Epicanthal folds, which represent a vertical fold of skin on either side of the nose sometimes covering the inner canthus, are seen as a facial characteristic in normal infants as well as in syndromes such as Down syndrome. In infants with Down syndrome the tongue may protrude, giving rise to the impression that macroglossia is present. In Down syndrome there is a short palate and, hence, this is a relative macroglossia.

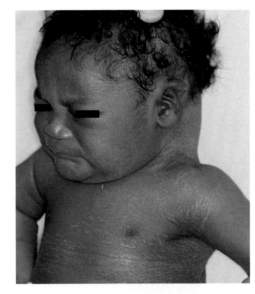

4.46

Figure 4.46. Webbing of the neck is a common finding in Down syndrome. This male infant with marked webbing of the neck and flat facies had the typical karyotype of trisomy 21. Because of the webbing, the neck may appear to be short.

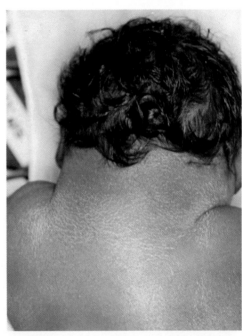

4.47

Figure 4.47. Posterior view of the same infant with trisomy 21 shows the marked webbing of the neck. Note that the hairline is high in contrast to Turner's syndrome where the hairline is low and the hair may be in whorls.

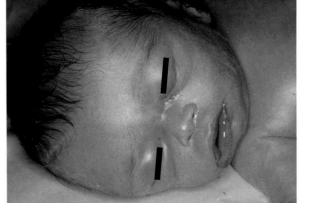

4.48

Figure 4.48. Down syndrome in a premature infant (gestational age of 33 weeks) with the typical karyotype of trisomy 21. The clinical diagnosis of Down syndrome may be difficult in small premature infants because the typical findings such as epicanthal folds, etc., are not as obvious as they are in the term infant.

4.49

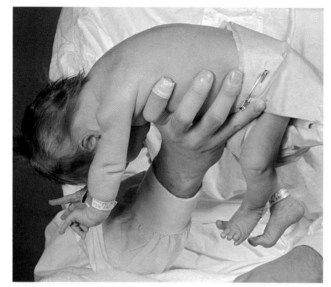

Figure 4.49. Marked hypotonia in an infant with Down syndrome. Hypotonia is present in over 80% of infants with Down syndrome. Also note the separation of the first and second toes.

4.50

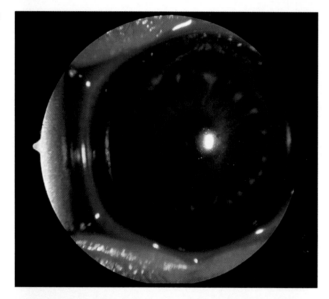

Figure 4.50. Brushfield's spots in the eyes of an infant with trisomy 21. These are aggregates of stromal fibers which form a ring around the iris near the limbus. They tend to disappear with age. Brushfield's spots may be seen in normal blue-eyed infants, but if present in infants with brown eyes they are pathologic. Brushfield's spots are also seen in infants with Zellweger syndrome.

4.51

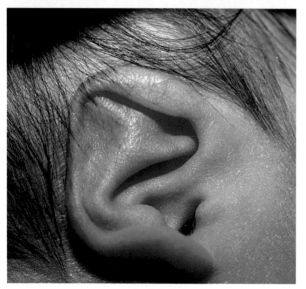

Figure 4.51. The typical square ("boxy") appearance of the ear in an infant with trisomy 21. Abnormalities of the ears are noted in at least 60% of infants with Down syndrome. Typically they are boxy, but they may be low set and small with overlapping of the helix and a prominent anthelix.

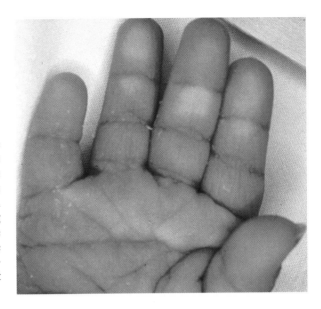

4.52

Figure 4.52. The typical short stubby fingers, single palmar (simian) crease, and clinodactyly of digit five on the right hand of an infant with trisomy 21. The short stubby fingers resulting in a short broad hand are noted in about 70% of infants with trisomy 21. A single palmar crease may be a normal variant occurring on both hands in 1 to 2% of the population and on one hand in 6%. Clinodactyly is incurving of the finger due to an absent or hypoplastic middle phalanx. Clinodactyly of the fifth digit is also seen as a normal variant and as a finding in many other syndromes.

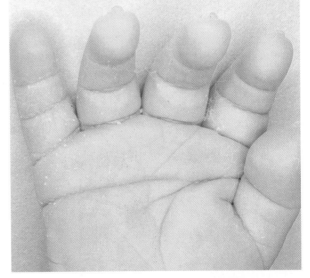

4.53

Figure 4.53. This infant with trisomy 21 has a single palmar crease. There is no clinodactyly but there is hypoplasia of the middle phalanx of the fifth finger as noted by the decreased distance between the finger creases. The single palmar crease is seen in about 45% of infants with trisomy 21 and is a finding in many other syndromes.

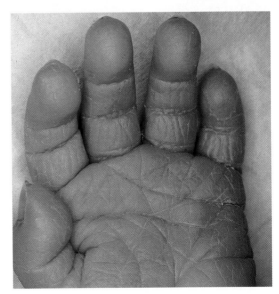

4.54

Figure 4.54. This infant with trisomy 21 has clinodactyly but normal palmar creases. Clinodactyly with an absent or hypoplastic middle phalanx of the fifth finger is present in about 50% of infants with trisomy 21.

4.55

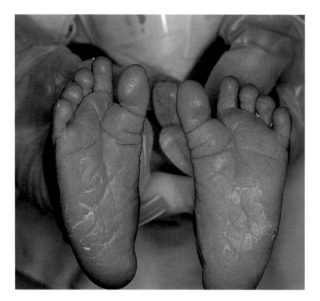

Figure 4.55. The gap between the first and second toes ("sandal" or "thong" sign) is a typical finding in trisomy 21. The feet are broad and short. The plantar surfaces are creased with a deep long furrow (ape-line) between the first and second toes.

4.56

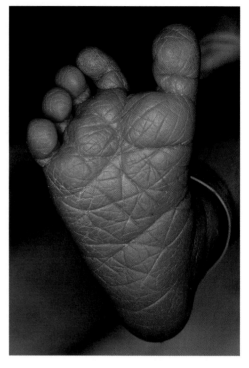

Figure 4.56. A close-up view of the broad short foot of an infant with trisomy 21 shows the marked separation of the first and second toes and the deep furrows on the sole.

4.57

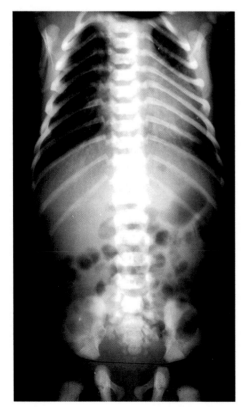

Figure 4.57. Total radiograph of an infant with trisomy 21 shows the long narrow chest cage with downslanting ribs due to hypotonia. Any infant who is hypotonic has this appearance of the chest cage. The finding of eleven pairs of ribs, as in this infant, is common in Down syndrome but also may occur as a finding in normal infants. The pelvis is a typical mongoloid pelvis. The infant also had congenital heart disease (the most common defect being an endocardial cushion defect).

4.58

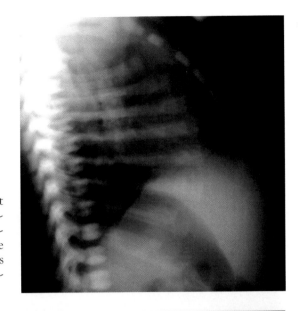

Figure 4.58. Lateral chest radiograph in another infant with trisomy 21 shows the increased number of sternal ossification centers. Compare this with trisomy 18 where ossification centers are decreased in number or absent (see Figure 4.36). Note that the ribs are normal in appearance as compared to the gracile delicate ribs seen in infants with trisomy 18.

4.59

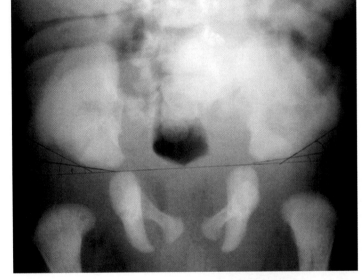

Figure 4.59. Radiograph of the typical mongoloid pelvis seen in infants with trisomy 21. Note the marked lateral flaring of the ilia giving rise to the so-called "Mickey Mouse" pelvis. There is a shallow acetabular angle. Compare this with the antimongoloid pelvis noted in infants with trisomy 18 (see Figure 4.37).

4.60

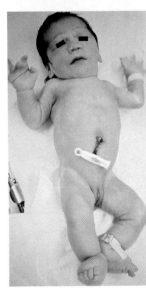

Figure 4.60. Infants with Turner's syndrome (XO syndrome) are phenotypically female although they have one of the pairs of X chromosomes missing. This term infant is short (length 43 cm) and demonstrates the short neck, shield-like chest with widely spaced nipples, and lymphedema, especially of the feet. Note also the single palmar crease on the right hand. Infants with Turner's syndrome may be small for gestational age.

4.61

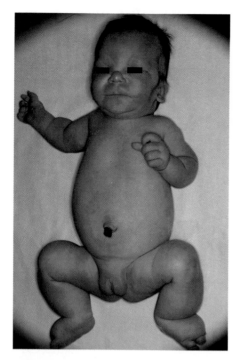

Figure 4.61. In another example of Turner's syndrome in a term infant (length 44 cm) note the marked lymphedema, especially of the lower extremities. Other findings in Turner's syndrome include a low posterior hairline with the appearance of a short neck, webbing of the neck, congenital heart disease (especially coarctation of the aorta), pigmented nevi, and skeletal abnormalities.

4.62

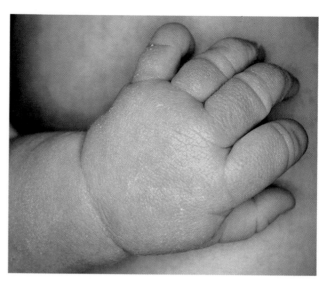

Figure 4.62. The same infant shows the marked lymphedema in the left hand. Transient congenital lymphedema with residual puffiness is noted over the dorsum of the hands and feet in more than 80% of infants with Turner's syndrome.

4.63

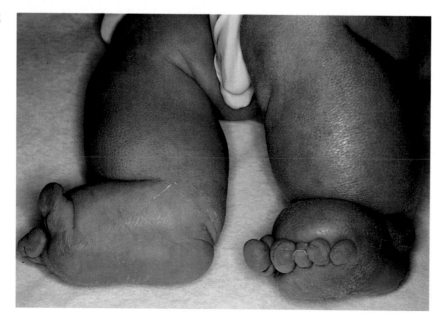

Figure 4.63. Note the hypoplastic nails in the same infant with Turner's syndrome. Hypoplastic finger and toe nails are commonly noted in infants with Turner's syndrome in that the nails are narrow, hyperconvex, and may be deep set.

4.64

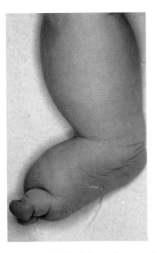
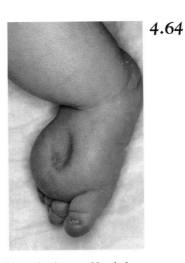

4.65

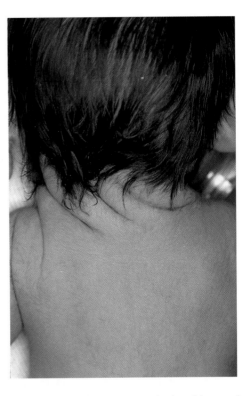

Figure 4.64. Note the marked lymphedema of both legs and feet in the same infant with Turner's syndrome. The marked lymphedema in Turner's syndrome is a pitting edema. Compare this with congenital lymphedema (Milroy's disease) where the edema is non-pitting.

Figure 4.65. There is marked webbing of the neck in this infant with Turner's syndrome. Note the low posterior hairline. Compare this with the webbing of the neck and high hairline in trisomy 21 (see Figure 4.47). The infant also had congenital heart disease (coarctation of the aorta).

4.66

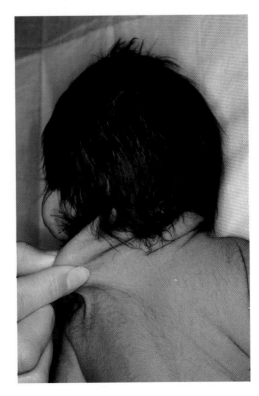

Figure 4.66. The marked webbing of the neck is again noted in this same infant with Turner syndrome. This results in the appearance of a shortened neck. The webbing of the neck occurs as a result of redundant skin.

A short neck may result from absence, malformation or coalescence of one or more cervical vertebrae, often giving the impression that the head is resting directly on the shoulders (Klippel-Feil syndrome, Jarcho-Levin syndrome). Neck webbing or high placement of the scapulae can give a similar appearance (Turner's syndrome, Down syndrome, cleidocranial dysostosis).

4.67

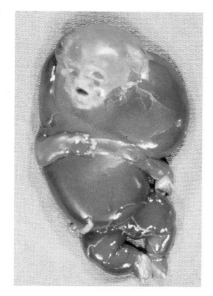

Figure 4.67. Fetal Turner's syndrome in an aborted fetus. Diagnosis was made prenatally by ultrasound and confirmed by karyotype. Note the large nuchal cystic hygromas of the neck and moderate hydrops of the limbs and body wall. This would explain the etiology of the redundant neck skin of these infants at birth. (R. Carpenter)

4.68

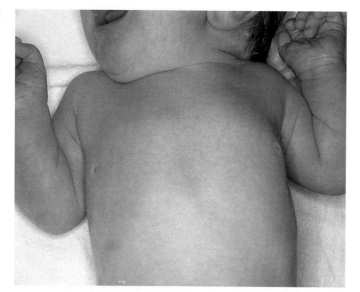

Figure 4.68. This infant with Turner's syndrome has the typical broad chest (shield-like chest) with widely spaced nipples. The nipples may be hypoplastic and/or inverted.

4.69

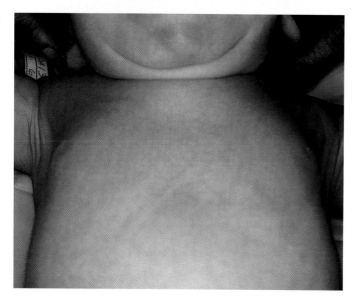

Figure 4.69. In Noonan's syndrome (Turner phenotype in the male) the typical findings are similar to those seen in Turner's syndrome. The infants are short in stature, have webbing of the neck, widely spaced nipples, lymphedema, and congenital heart disease (especially pulmonic stenosis). In this male infant with Noonan's syndrome note the shield-like chest and widely spaced nipples.

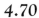

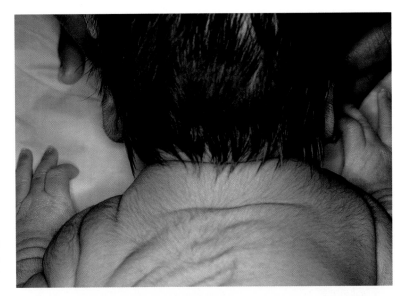

Figure 4.70. The same infant has the typical appearance of a short neck, redundant skin, and low posterior hairline.

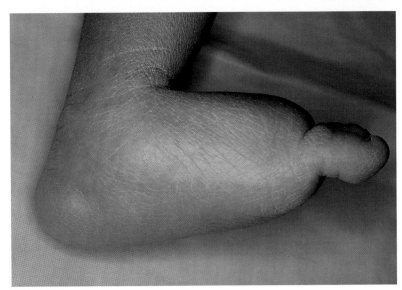

Figure 4.71. Lymphedema of the dorsum of the foot in the same infant with Noonan's syndrome.

Index

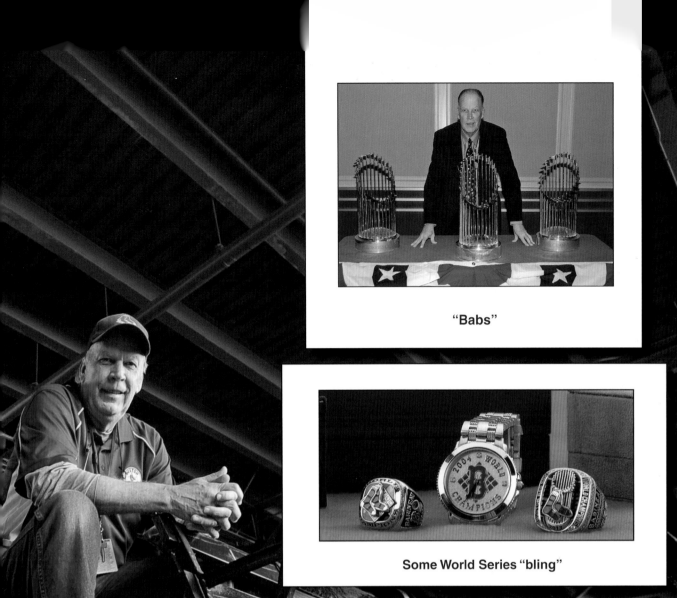

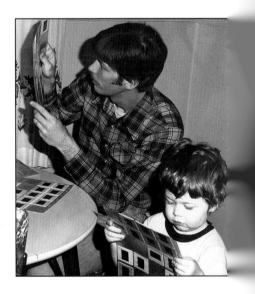

"Babs"

Some World Series "bling"

"Babs"

Steve, Chris Babineau